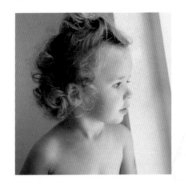

BABY BODY LANGUAGE

100 WAYS TO UNDERSTAND BABIES & TODDLERS

EMMA HOWARD

COLLINS & BROWN

First published in the United Kingdom in 2008 by
Salamander Books,
A division of the Pavilion Books Company Ltd.
43 Great Ormond Street, London WC1N 3HZ

Distributed in the United States and Canada by
Sterling Publishing Co., Inc.
1166 Avenue of the Americas
New York, NY 10036, USA

All notations of errors or omissions should be addressed to Salamander Books,
43 Great Ormond Street, London WC1N 3HZ

ISBN: 978-1-911163-51-0

Printed in China

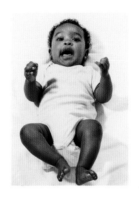

BABY BODY LANGUAGE

100 WAYS TO UNDERSTAND BABIES & TODDLERS

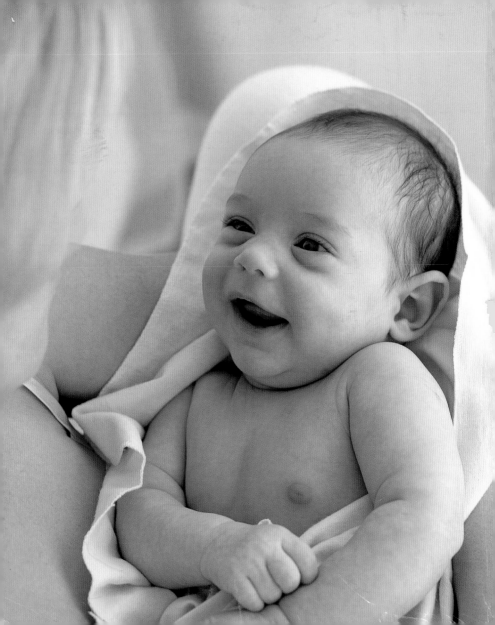

CONTENTS

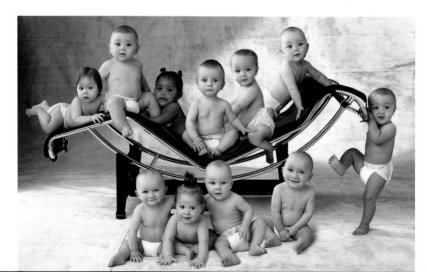

INTRODUCTION

For decades, experts have studied the importance of nonverbal communication in adults. The idea that the body has its own innate language has become so accepted in our society that magazines and newspapers regularly print articles on how to read and interpret those hidden signals we all send out. It is universally acknowledged that adults use body language, both consciously and unconsciously. Studies have shown that up to 60 percent of all human interaction is based not on speech but on the subtle movements, gestures, and responses of our bodies. This includes the tiniest reactions, such as the dilation of the pupils or a slightly increased rate of breathing, to the more obvious signals like smiling, frowning, and establishing personal space.

Surprisingly, babies are experts on the use and understanding of body language, as they have no other means of communication. Until they learn to talk, children are completely dependent on body language, and even after they have mastered speaking, their actions still play a massive role in their communication skills. They may not have the words to express themselves, but they always manage to get their points across. Whether summoning attention through tears or smiles, a baby can always make its wants and needs known.

For parents with new babies—whether their first child or fourth—life would be much less frustrating if they could understand exactly what their infant is trying to express. Indeed, a child's cries can become a major source of concern. Although we try our best to comfort small children, sometimes there is just no knowing what a child is trying to tell us and we are left to run through a checklist of possibilities: Is she uncomfortable? Hungry? Tired? Scared? This is when understanding and interpreting your baby's body language can become

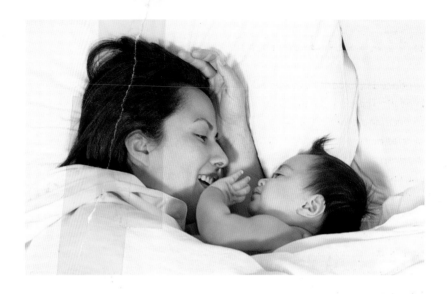

extremely helpful.

From newborns to toddlers, children use a wide variety of gestures and actions to communicate with the adults around them. Indeed, without them, caring for a child would be extremely difficult. As parents, many of our responses are completely instinctive, though often correct. Few mothers can stand still for long once they hear the distinctive cry of distress from their own child. Any parent would find it difficult not to smile back at a young baby when he or she smiles at you. From the moment it enters the world, everything a baby does helps to ensure he or she is looked after and protected by his or her parents. There are powerful biological, hormonal, and physical imperatives all urging us on to cherish and care for the small, helpless child in front of us. It is our duty as parents and caregivers to provide a loving, nurturing home, to give our children a sense of self-worth and confidence, and also to show them the importance of understanding. We expect them to listen to what we say, and to do this we show them how gratifying it is when they are listened to and understood. By learning to interpret your child's body language, you will better understand their motivations and thought processes, and instill in them the idea that you empathize and understand them. Few things are more important to a child.

Studying your baby's body language will not only help you to better know your child, but will help you to appreciate how your own actions can encourage, or possibly hinder, your child's development. For example, when feeding a child solid food for the first time, most people will unconsciously

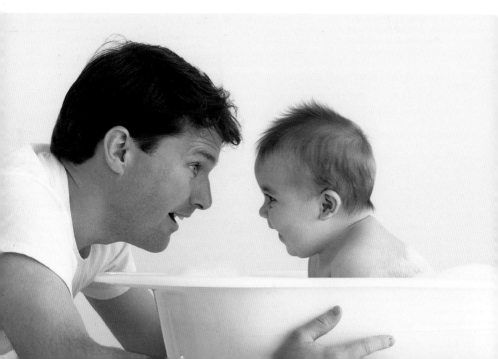

open and close their mouths, make "num-num" noises, and demonstrate the action of swallowing. All these simple gestures teach children more than just actions; they also teach the appropriate reactions. Children who are taught to understand, learn from, and respond to the body language of others will become more confident and easygoing adults. We learn our social skills from the examples set by others, usually our parents. With this in mind, you should remember to pay close attention to your own body language. Babies learn quickly, and unfortunately, they pick up both good and bad habits. If you can provide a good role model for your child by using positive body language, it will help your child to develop into a self-assured and confident adult. A baby not only discovers how to use his or her own body language to interact with the people around him or her, but quickly learns to interpret the gestures of others. As babies quickly grow into toddlers, they learn to combine their body language with their rudimentary language skills, and should they glean any negative habits from you, these will soon become apparent. Toddlers love to impersonate the behavior of those closest to them; it is how they learn to be adults, and should any of your less admirable practices come back to haunt you, you have only yourself to blame.

Raising a child is a wonderful, exciting, testing, tiring, and joyful pursuit. There are few times in your life that will cause you to laugh quite so often or enjoy life quite so much. By studying the nonverbal communications of your infant, you will not be able to read minds. However, it will give you a better understanding of how your child really feels, why he or she does certain things, and what these actions mean. Anything that helps you to feel closer to and empathize with your child is well worth exploring.

01

"I'M COMPLETELY ADORABLE."

Although totally vulnerable at birth, babies actually have an arsenal of "parent-trapping weapons" at their disposal. Even their simple presence induces an "ahhh factor" in adults that virtually guarantees they will be cared for and loved. Their large eyes set low in the face, high foreheads, chubby little arms and legs, all promote a strong nurturing instinct in adults, particularly in women.

KNEES, PLEASE

When they are first born, babies don't have kneecaps. They develop in the latter half of the child's first year. Also, babies enter the world with 300 bones in their bodies, where adults have only 206. This is because many of the bones fuse together as the child becomes older.

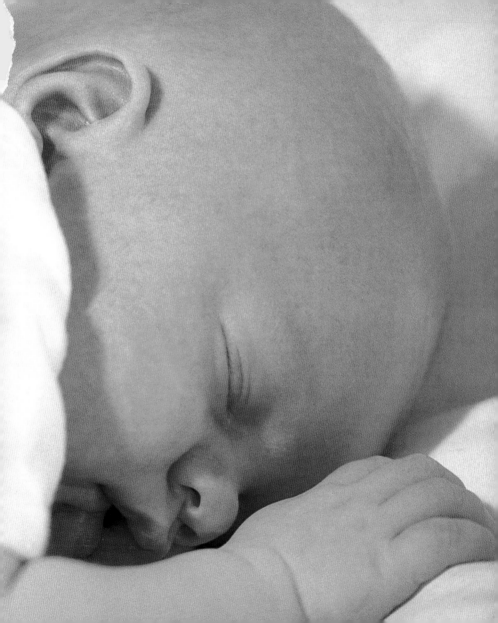

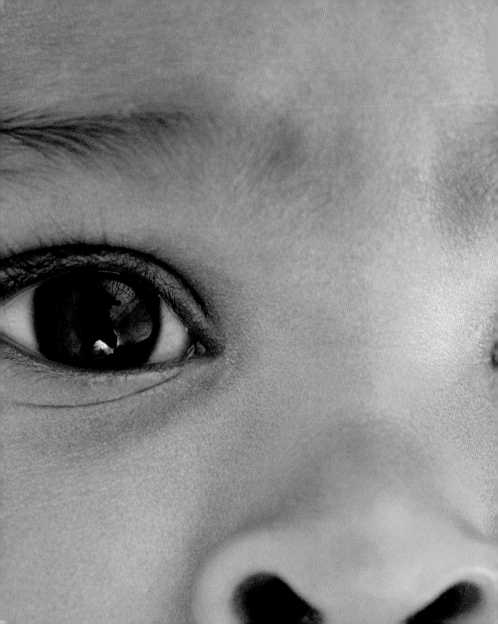

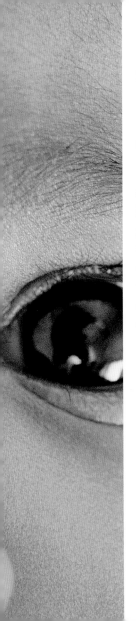

02

"WHAT BIG EYES I HAVE!"

One of the most powerful yet often unnoticed forms of baby body language is dilation of the pupils. The larger the pupils become, the higher the regard. A baby's pupils are much larger than normal and therefore the reaction is more conspicuous. By widely opening their eyes and focusing on the object in sight—usually a parent—a young child not only takes in more but gives the parent a sense that they are accepted and adored. This further strengthens the bond between carer and child.

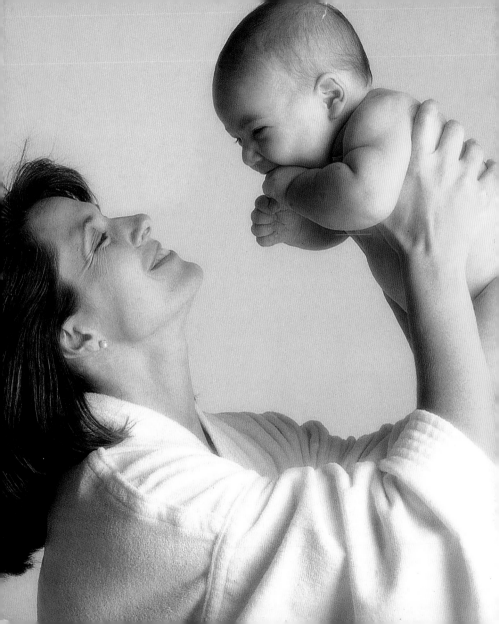

03 "I GOTCHA."

Not all of a newborn baby's responses are an attempt at communication; many of a baby's actions just after birth are purely instinctive. For example, when a baby is startled, she will throw out her arms and legs. She will turn her head when someone touches her cheek, or grab a finger when someone strokes her palm. All babies are born with these reflexes and over time they will disappear.

THE "MORO REFLEX"

The "Moro reflex"—or a baby's action of throwing out her arms and legs when falling—is thought to be an evolutionary throwback from when we were apes. When a baby feels herself falling, she responds in exactly the same way as an infant ape, reaching out for the safety of her mother's fur. The reflex is common to all babies at birth but gradually fades over the following weeks, completely disappearing by the age of two months.

04 "BIRD? WHERE? AND WHAT'S A BIRD ANYWAY?"

You may notice there are times when the eyes of your child become crossed or appear not to be working together. This is not a cause for alarm. When first born, the eyes of a newborn are only strong enough to see clearly for a short distance—usually between seven and twelve inches—approximately the distance from the mother's breast to her baby's face. When babies try to focus on anything farther away, their eye muscles are not strong enough to cope and this causes them to go out of unison. It should fade with time as the eye muscles become stronger.

HAZARDS? WHAT HAZARDS?

There is a good reason why babies can't see very far—it is an efficient guard against unnecessary stress. If newborns, in their vulnerable and weak state, could see the world around them and all the potential threats they may face, it would cause them severe anxiety. They don't actually need to see any farther than the face of their mother.

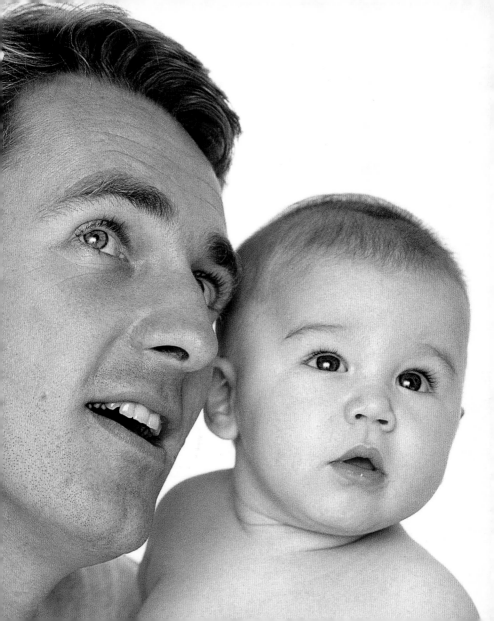

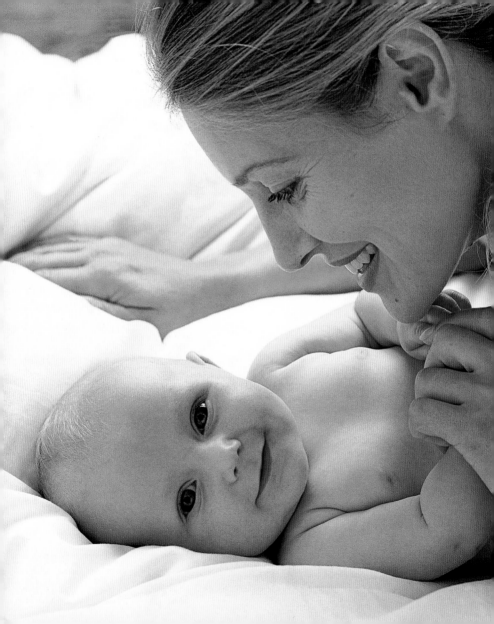

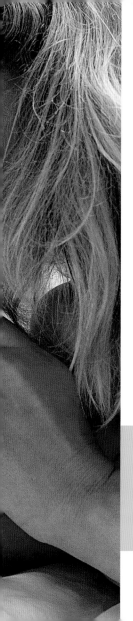

05

"I CAN HEAR SO MUCH."

We know that babies begin to respond to sounds while still in the womb. A baby can differentiate between many different sounds and can distinguish the sound of their mother's voice from other female voices within the first week of life. A newborn baby cannot turn his head toward the sound to show recognition, but he does move his eyes. In a test to prove newborns could pinpoint and recognize different sounds, a baby was put in a room and his mother put in a soundproof booth, positioned right in front of the child. Only when the mother's face was combined with her voice coming from the same direction did the infant appear happy and not distressed.

WHERE'S THAT BAT?

A baby can hear sounds as low as sixteen cycles per second and as high as 20,000 cycles per second. Adult ears are not as efficient. The lower sounds remain stable but the older we get, the harder it is to hear higher-pitched noises.

06 "TWO HOURS OLD AND I'M BORED ALREADY."

Just after birth, a baby will often take several huge yawns. It is natural to suppose that he is tired after such an exhausting commute down the birth canal. The real reason is that these yawns are a reflex action and allow the brand-new, never-before-used lungs to take in large amounts of much-needed oxygen.

SOUL MEANS OF ESCAPE

According to the superstitions of ancient Rome, yawning was seen as a foreteller of doom. When babies yawned it was thought that a piece of their soul escaped through their open mouths. Mothers were encouraged to cover the yawn with their hands in order to halt this "deterioration" of the soul.

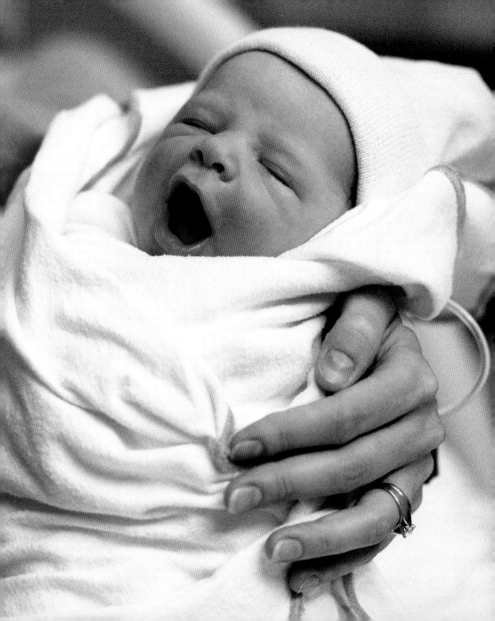

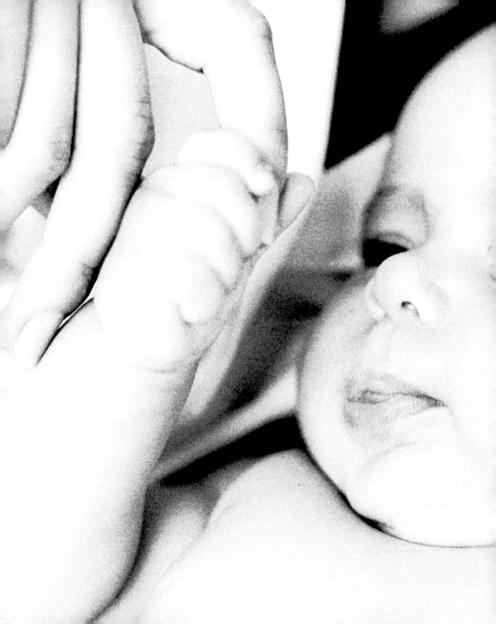

07

"I MIGHT LET GO . . .
I MIGHT NOT."

When first born, a baby will often keep its hands tightly clenched or wrapped tightly around any finger within reach. This is an instinctive response and will fade in time. As they grow, children become more in control of their movements and young infants are often fascinated with their own hands. By watching your child's hands, it is possible to read their mood. For example, a relaxed and happy child will have relaxed and open hands.

GET A GRIP

The grasping reflex in newborn babies is surprisingly strong. The grip can be so firm that it is possible to lift the baby in the air. Although it is tempting to test this particular reflex, a word of warning. As with most instinctive newborn reactions, this fades very quickly.

08 "YOU SMELL FAMILIAR."

A newborn baby is quickly able to distinguish the shape, sound, and even smell of her parents, singling them out with smiles or just watching them intently, even when surrounded by other adults. These simple signs of recognition can be extremely gratifying to parents and foster understandable feelings of pride and joy. Following these subtle signs of a child's approval, parents will often reward her with smiles, cuddles, and praise—thus making her feel loved in return and encouraging her to continue with this form of communication.

THE RIGHT SNIFF

One little-known fact about a newborn's sense of smell is how quickly it can learn to distinguish the smell of its mother from that of any other woman. If the new mother and child remain in close contact after the delivery, then within forty-five hours the newborn will recognize and single out its mother purely by her smell.

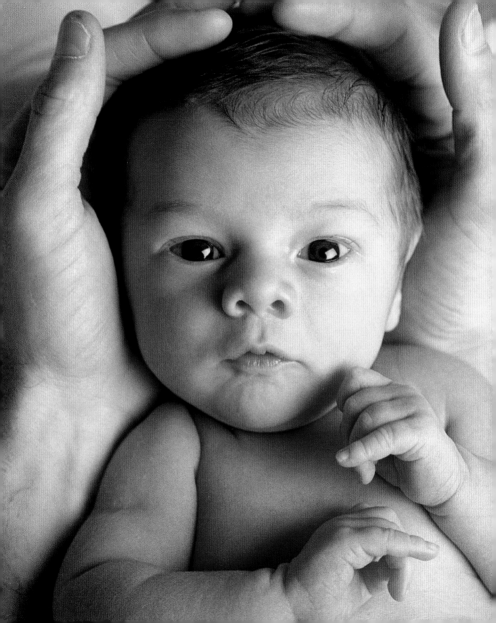

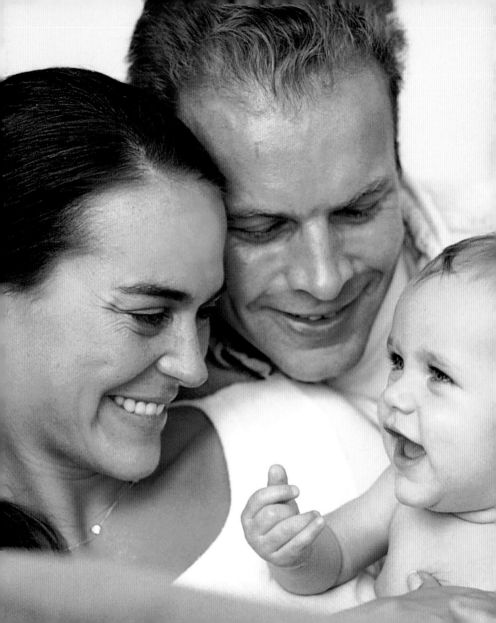

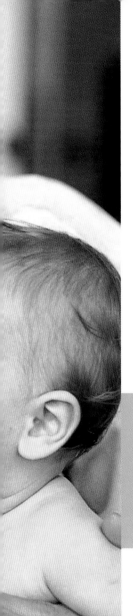

09

"YOU TWO LOOK FAMILIAR."

From as young as eight weeks old, babies can recognize different people and will respond. Studies have shown that babies can recognize the faces of their parents as quickly as two or three weeks after birth. Although more receptive to the well-loved faces of its parents, young babies do not display "stranger anxiety" until around six months old. With strangers, a baby of that age will often make noises of discomfort, and will look for the reassuring sight of their mother.

THE FACE FITS

New forms of testing have proven that babies recognize the faces of their parents much earlier than previously thought (three to four months). When photos were combined with the sounds of the parents' voices, the baby exhibited excitement and recognition.

10

"HEY, BIG DADDY."

Soon after birth, a baby will recognize the sound of her mother's (and father's) voice, and will turn her head toward the sound. Before long she will begin to mimic the facial expressions of her parents in the first steps toward interaction; opening and closing her mouth, putting out her tongue, and smiling. All these actions are important because they promote a bond between child and parent—after all, mimicry is the highest form of flattery. Typically, a newborn baby takes just seven days to recognize the sound of her mother's voice, and fourteen days to memorize the sound of her father's.

SOUNDS FAMILIAR

Babies become familiar with the distinctive tones of their parents while still in the womb. Studies have shown that when fetuses hear either their mother's or father's voice, their heart rate will quicken, but when listening to a stranger's voice, the heart rate decelerates.

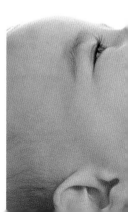

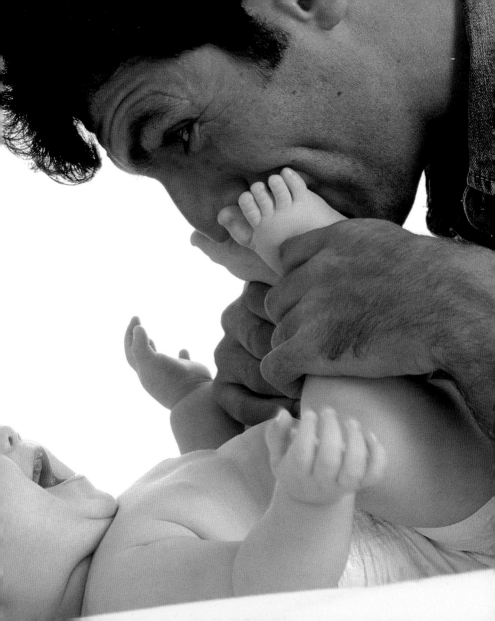

11

"I LIKE YOU—YOU'VE GOT FOOD."

When first born, a baby can only focus within a few inches. However, infants can recognize a human face almost immediately. The attraction of newborn children to faces is thought to play a key role in the mother and baby bonding process. While a mother is breast-feeding her new baby, their faces are only a few inches apart—the ideal distance for the baby to become familiar. Fathers can also experience this same bonding process while bottle-feeding.

SWITCHED ON FROM BIRTH

For the first hour after birth, babies are more alert than they will be for the following few days, when they will spend most of their time sleeping. If given the chance, the newborn will spend this hour gazing attentively at his mother's face, a valuable time of bonding.

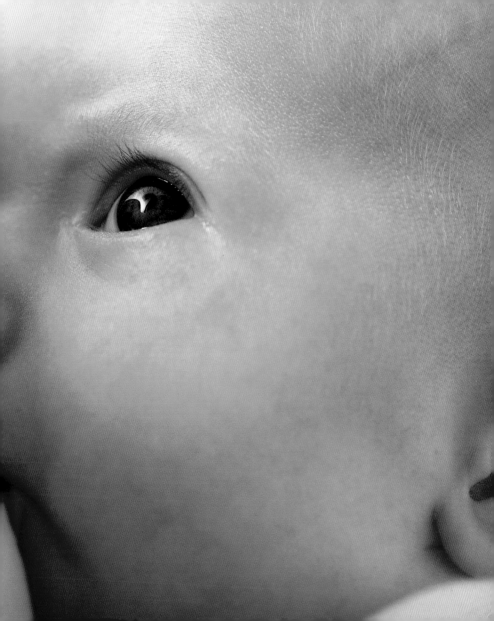

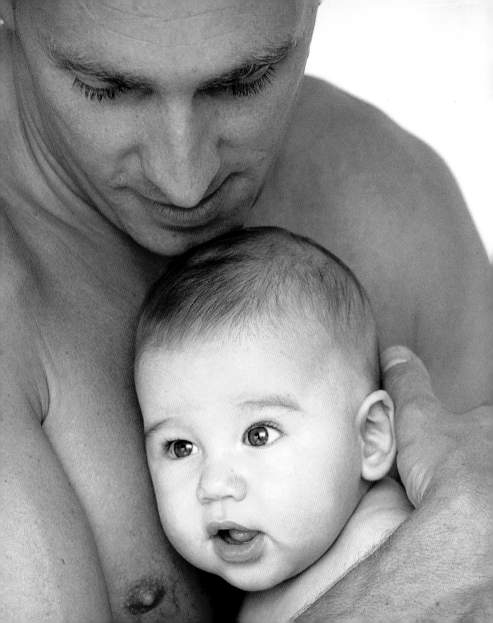

12 "NOW IT'S QUALITY TIME WITH DAD."

Bath time with dad is an important part of a baby's development. A fourteen-year study by a London psychologist has reported that babies who miss out on being bathed by their fathers have a far greater risk of developing social problems in later life. The study revealed that 30% of boys and girls who were not bathed regularly by their father were likely to have "significant friendship problems" when they grew up.

13 "WHEE! THIS IS FUN!"

Playing with babies is rewarding for both the parents and the child, but it is often difficult to tell whether you are sparking your child's interest. When fascinated by something or someone, a baby will display their curiosity using a number of instinctive actions. A younger child will try to reach up to the object of their fascination, and if they have not yet mastered the use of their limbs, their arms may wave about excitedly. They will open and close their fists in an attempt to grab. If very excited, their legs will kick out spasmodically as the enthusiasm becomes too much to bear. All these actions are signs that your child is interested and enjoying the game.

THE CRYING GAME

Studies have shown that as soon as two days after the birth, 50 percent of mothers could distinguish their baby's particular "distressed" cry from a group of thirty other children.

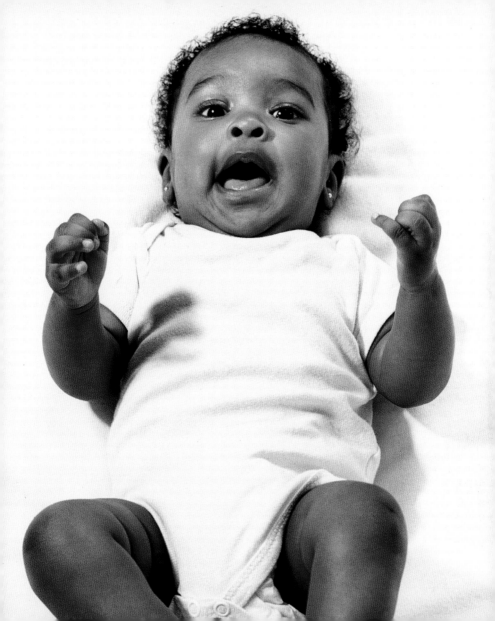

14

"THIS TASTES OKAY TO PLAY WITH."

Toddlers and older children will show whether they are interested in a toy or game in a more measured and much calmer way than young babies. They will lean forward to take a closer look, often reaching out to touch or even taste the object of fascination. They may be intently silent, staring at the item and just taking it all in. Also they might sit with their legs folded underneath them. This position, even in adults, shows curiosity.

LISTENING IN

As they reach six months old, children will begin to pay attention to the sounds of entire words. Rhythm in speech will help them to memorize more common words. In fact, the more words a baby hears, the more she will understand.

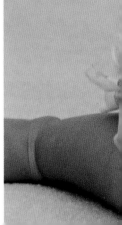

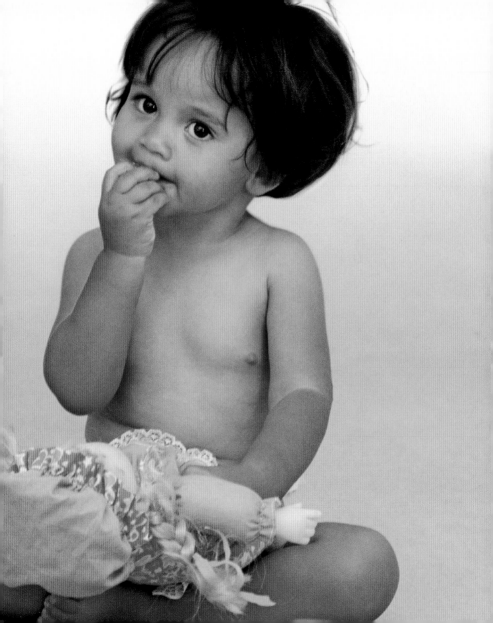

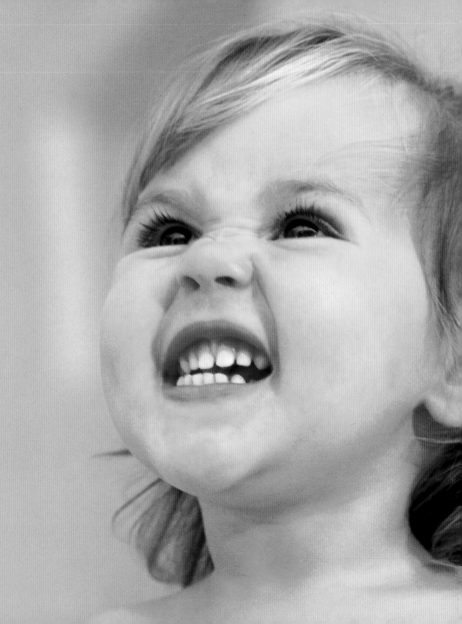

15 "MOM, THIS ONE'S REALLY EASY."

It has happened to all parents at one time or another. Your child has dropped her toy and wants you to get it back for her; she may even point at it and shout. No sooner do you give it back to her than she throws it on the ground again, continuing her demands that you pick it up. Believe it or not, she is not trying to be irritating; she is playing with you. She has made up a game all by herself and wants you to join in. The title of this game could be "make mommy really tired" but it is a milestone in your child's comprehension of the world. She is learning about cause and effect—by throwing the toy, mommy bends down to get it—and also learning to make herself understood through signals like pointing and shouting.

DON'T MAKE ME LAUGH

On average, a six-year-old will laugh 300 times every day. Adults seem gloomy in comparison, only laughing sixty times per day.

16

"NICE TRY, BUT I PREFER THE MOBILE."

The first form of play involves the excitement babies experience while watching the movement of interesting shapes. A newborn's eyes are not yet fully developed, so it takes a few weeks for this game to really catch on, normally at about two months old. An interesting mobile hung over the crib will keep a baby fascinated for a long time. At this early stage of life, a baby is enthralled by any moving shapes that cross its field of vision. As with all games, they will become boring without variation.

TOYS-AREN'T-US

During the first year of life, a baby will have little use for toys. It is not until the second year that more sophisticated playthings will become of interest. For the first twelve months, a baby's ideal plaything will be his parents.

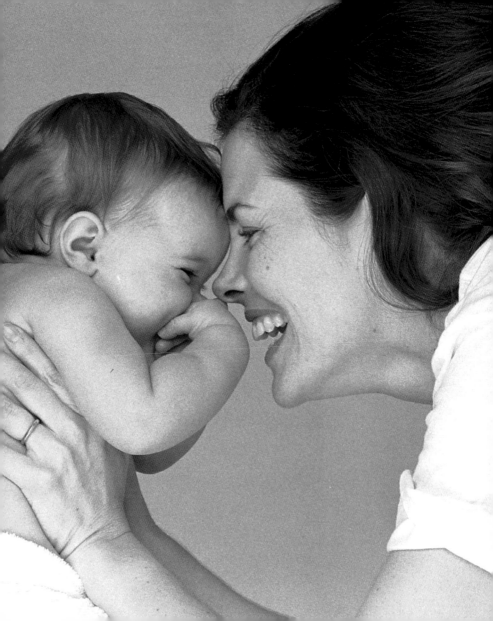

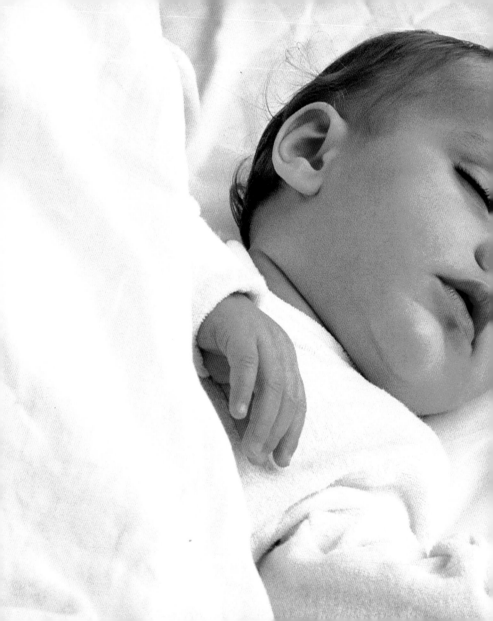

17

"I COULD USE A NAP."

For a parent, it is important to be able to read the moods of your child. By watching and remembering the telltale clues, you should be able to predict their patterns and therefore settle them into a routine more easily. Learning to tell when they are tired is extremely important because a baby denied sleep will become fussy, making it all the more difficult to get them to sleep. Drooping eyelids, blinking slowly, or stiff, erratic movements are classic signals of fatigue in babies. When children get slightly older, they may become irritable, overexcited, or extra clingy.

GIVE IT A REST

It is almost impossible to communicate properly with a tired child. Babies are much more receptive to you while alert. Choose a time of day when your child will be bright and active, and talk to her quietly and rhythmically using lots of facial expressions and sounds.

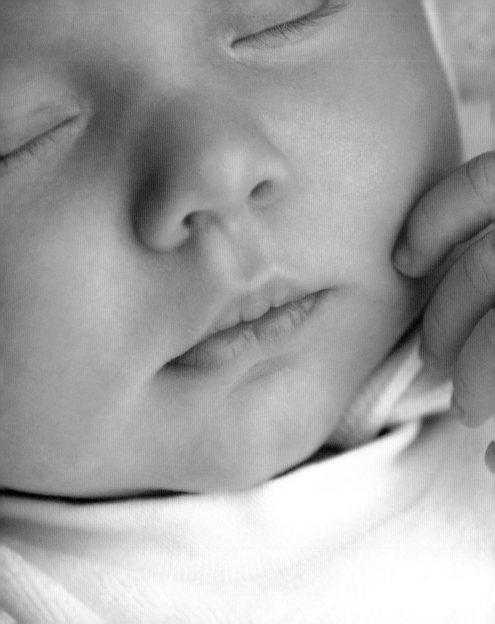

18

"THAT'S BETTER."

One of the most indicative signs that your baby is tired is when she starts rubbing her eyes. Most babies will scrunch up their eyes and rub their curled fists over their eyelids when sleepy. It is a universal signal that it is time for a nap. Why eye rubbing in particular? As babies get tired, the muscles in their eyes become sore, and just like when an adult uses a particular muscle too much, it will become tender. Rubbing relieves this discomfort. It also encourages the tear ducts to begin producing moisture, as tired eyes are often hot and dry.

HA! FOOLED YOU!

Just to confuse you, babies love experimenting with every part of their bodies. It could be that they are simply rubbing their closed eyes because when they do, they can see flashing lights and colors.

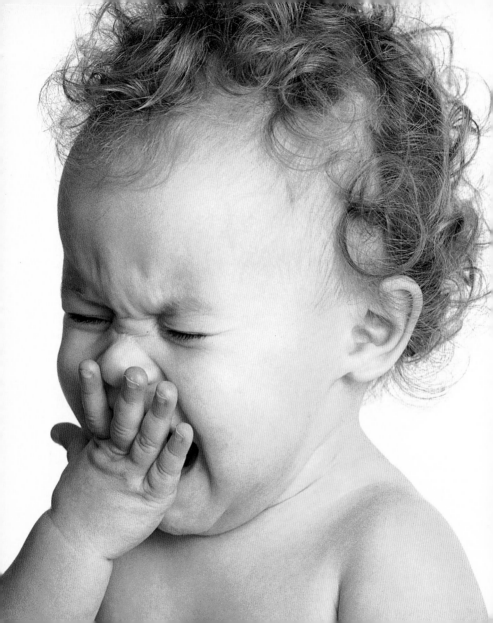

19 "I DON'T WANT TO MISS OUT ON ANYTHING."

Whether firstborn or six months old, most children will go through a difficult phase of resisting sleep. This is a grueling time for sleep-deprived parents as their bundle of joy forces herself to stay awake despite the late hour. Babies resist going to sleep for two main reasons: The first is that now they are in this exciting, sensory-rich world, they do not want to leave it for something as dull as sleep. The second reason is they do not want to be parted from their parents.

THE BIGGEST TEDDIES

Babies in cultures where children and parents sleep together are rarely upset or resist bedtime. They go to bed calmly and are lulled to sleep by the rhythmic sound of a nearby adult's breathing.

20 "TEDDY'S COMING TO BED—OR ELSE."

Many young children become overattached to objects such as a security blanket, a favorite plush toy, or a pacifier. Sometimes the attachment is so strong that the child becomes upset if parted from it, and is then unable to sleep. These objects are acting as a replacement for physical contact with parents. These "security objects" provide the child with a constant and readily available companion who is always ready to receive and, in their own way, give affection. There has been much discussion as to whether these items are good for children or should be avoided. The most important point should be the comfort of the child. If for some reason it is impossible for the parents to give as much physical contact as the baby requires, the appearance of a security object can be a welcome relief.

BLANKET COVERAGE

Tests have shown that children who have not bonded well with their mothers but who have a security blanket deal much better with stressful and anxious situations than those without a security blanket.

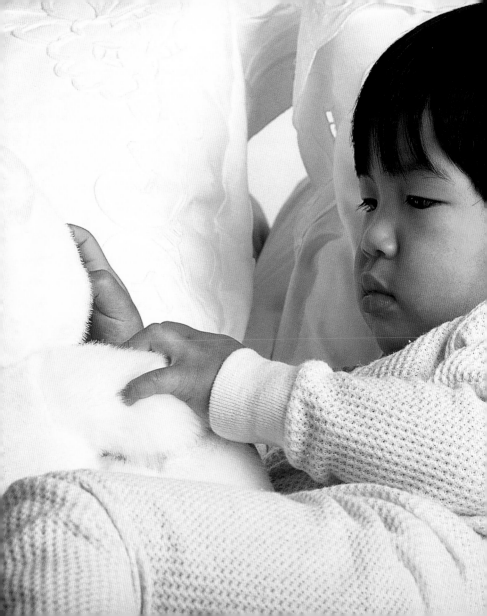

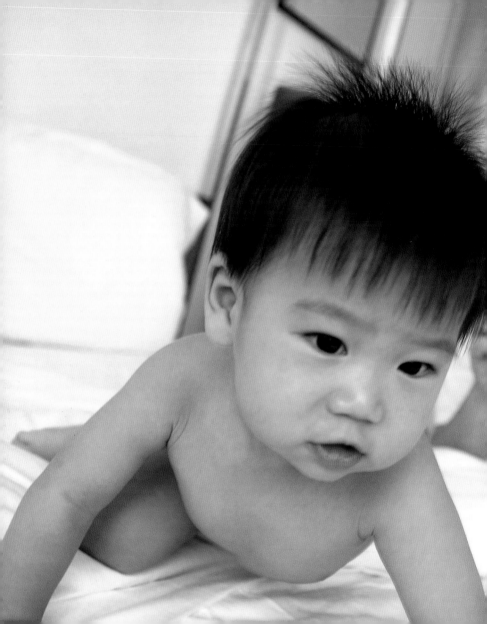

21

"I'M OUTTA HERE!"

Around two years old, your child will move from sleeping in a crib to sleeping in a "grown-up" bed. It is a huge milestone in their life and a reminder to you of how quickly time flies. However, it can also be a difficult time when trying to get them to stay in the new bed. No longer surrounded by protective bars, your child will find it very easy to get out of bed. Toddlers are naturally curious and love your company, so if they can come and find you—they will!

ROUTINE MAINTENANCE

To promote a calm bedtime, it is important to give your baby a bedtime routine—washing, brushing teeth, bedtime stories, and a kiss goodnight will all help calm her to sleep. If she does continue to get up, just take her back to bed as quickly as possible and without talking to her. They will quickly learn that bedtime means sleep time.

"I COULD DO THIS FOR HOURS."

You may notice your baby's eyes move while she is asleep. Sometimes this is accompanied by giggles or smiles. The rapid eye movements (or REM) indicate when babies are dreaming. The average baby will sleep for 16.6 hours every day during the first week after birth. By a month old, this will drop to 14.8 hours a day and continues to decline until the child is a year old. The average toddler will sleep for 12 hours a day.

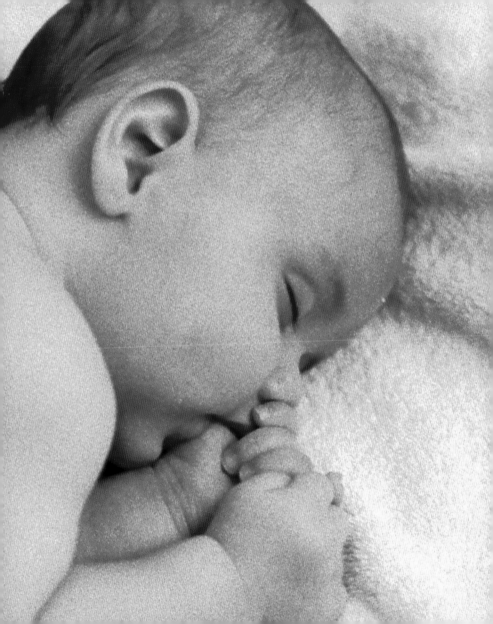

23

"I'M HAPPY."

There are few things more rewarding or heartwarming as
your baby's first smile. It is something you remember for the
rest of your life. Younger babies, up to a month old, are often
seen giving a lopsided, almost drunken smile when they need
burping, and sometimes they will smile when surprised by a
voice or a tickle. This "reflex smile" is the first stage of smiling
in babies and is more of an instinctive reaction rather than a
true smile.

SMILE IF YOU MEAN IT

Human beings are the only creatures on the planet who
use smiling as a form of communication and approbation.
To us, it is a signal of friendliness and salutation throughout
the world, but for the rest of the animals on the planet, the
baring of teeth is interpreted as a sign of aggression and
challenge.

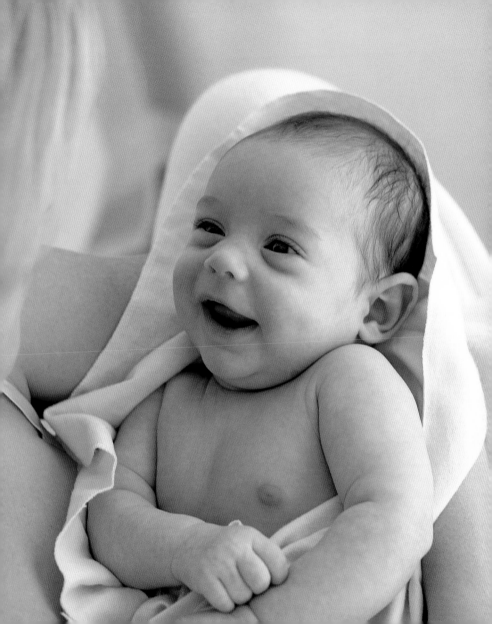

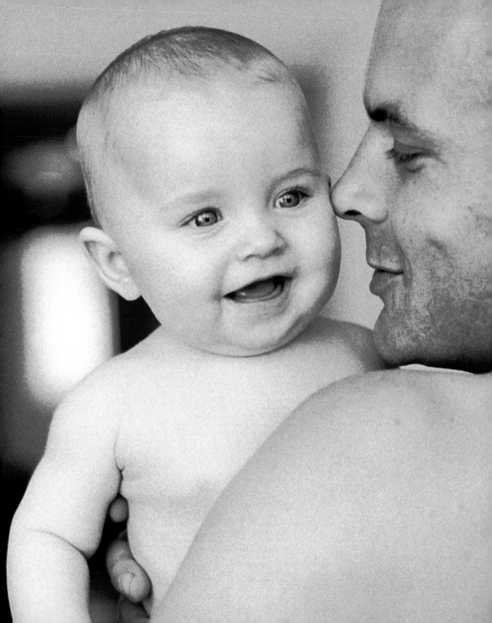

24 "I'LL SMILE AT ANYONE"

The next stage in smiling is known as the "general smile." At around four weeks old your baby will have mastered the art of smiling and will often give wide, delighted, gummy grins. This is extremely gratifying for parents, but at this stage a baby will probably respond this way to any adult face it sees. By now, a baby knows the act of smiling is important but has yet to realize that it is crucial to discern at what or whom it smiles.

NATAL TEETH

One out of every 2,000 babies is born with a tooth already showing. These early teeth are called "natal teeth" and usually only one will appear at the front of the mouth, though in very rare cases there are two teeth visible. The natal teeth are poorly rooted and will wobble around freely in the gum. This is fortunate, as they won't hinder breast-feeding.

25 "NOW YOU—YOU'RE FUNNY."

The final stage of smiling is called the "specific smile" and this is the smile parents wait impatiently for. Between four and six months old, a baby will begin to reserve his smiles for only those people close to him. The big, open smiles are now only for his parents or close contacts. Strangers, who perhaps a few weeks ago were greeted by the nonspecific "general smile," will now find themselves shunned and even screamed at. This can be a very rewarding feeling for parents—who may feel as though they have entered an exclusive club and have been ushered into the VIP room.

NO FAKE SMILES

Of course, adults have an additional stage of smiling, which is the diplomatic smile—a form of general smile often used despite their true feelings. Babies are above such duplicity and will scream at any unwelcome guests. If only grown-ups could do this, too.

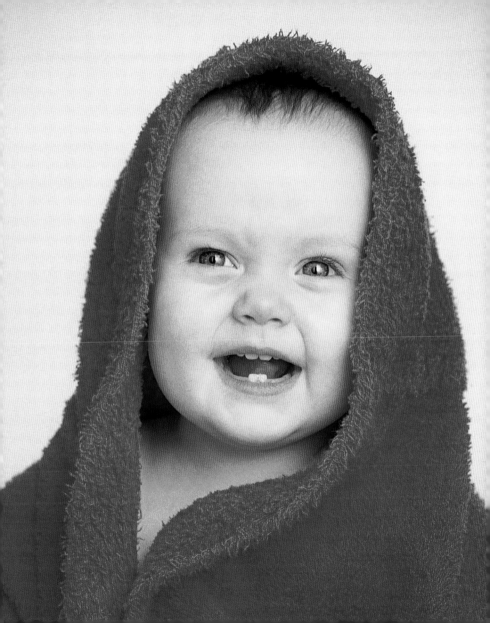

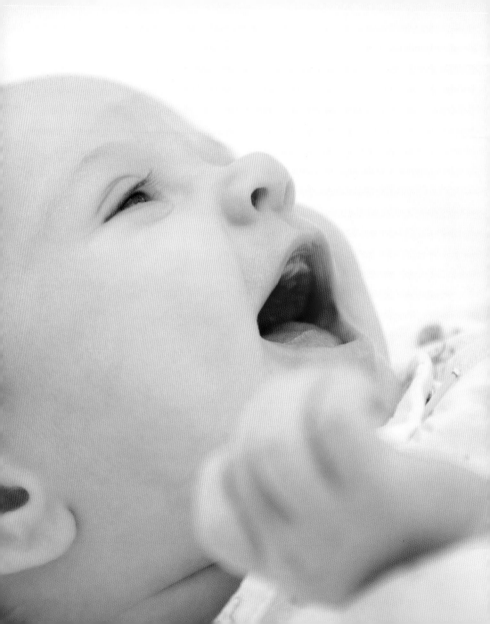

26 "I LOVE THE CUSTARD PIE GAG! AGAIN, AGAIN!"

As a parent, few things are more infectious and wonderful than your child's first laugh. What makes babies—and for that matter, adults—laugh has forever been a subject of debate. An infant's first laugh usually happens after she has learned to recognize the differences between her mother and other female adults. Sometimes it begins with an unexpected "Boo!" or a funny face from grandad, or it could be a more boisterous game of tickles or "flying" when she is held high in the air like an airplane. All of a sudden the joyful giggle pops out. The one thing all these games have in common is a sense of danger combined with the safety that a parent represents. She knows her mother would never do anything bad to her, so she is relaxed enough to enjoy the shock and turns it into laughter.

LAUGHTER IS THE BEST MEDICINE

Some scientists believe that the laughter shared between parent and child when playing tickle games helps promote bonding. It also teaches the baby that laughing feels good, which encourages more giggles.

27

"STOP THIS! TAKE IT AWAY, NOW!"

A newborn's cry is always a signal of distress and should be attended to quickly. Babies cry for many reasons, the main ones being pain, hunger, discomfort, loneliness, frustration, overstimulation, and understimulation. Although the problem is not always immediately obvious to the parent, sometimes just the simple act of his protector arriving will be enough to calm a crying child. It is important to remember that however frustrated you may become trying to find the source of your child's distress, newborns never use crying to express themselves in an attempt to unleash pent-up emotion.

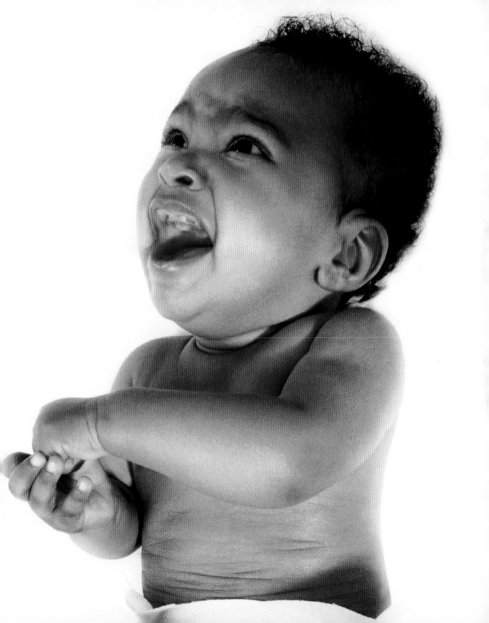

28 "WHERE'S EVERYBODY GONE?"

Parents are often surprised to discover that loneliness is one of the major reasons their baby starts to cry. Years of evolution have programmed babies to crave the company and physical contact of their parents, so tears often arrive when they are denied this primal need. Without the touch or closeness of a parent or protector, babies can feel isolated and insecure and will often cry until back in the calming environment of their mother's arms. This can be inconvenient for today's modern, busy, and often stressed parent, but there are times when only a hug will do.

PAIN OR MISERY?

Mothers who have bonded with their newborns will also become adept at understanding the many different types of crying. Not all cries are the heartbreaking, earth-shattering sobs of real pain or distress, and mothers will soon learn to detect the different tones. When awakened by a howl of pain, her reactions are much faster than at any other time.

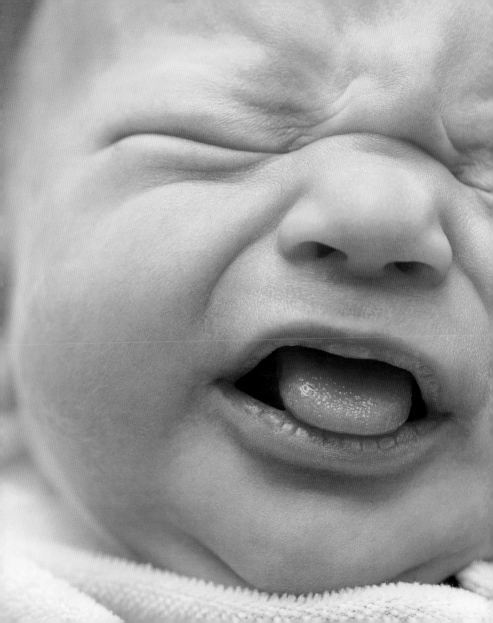

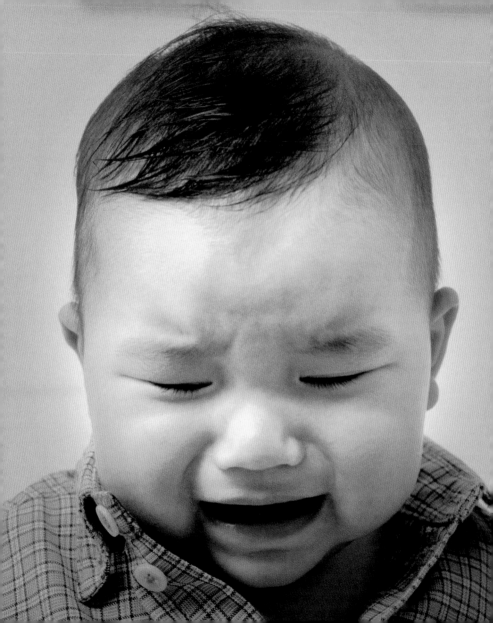

29 "I WAS HUNGRY, BUT NOW I'M ANGRY!"

A child that cries from hunger often gets into such a state of distress that even when offered the food it so desperately wants, such as the breast or bottle, it has become too agitated to drink it. This can be incredibly upsetting for the parents as they try to give their infant what it needs, but are unable to stop them crying long enough so they can begin to suck. In situations like this, where the baby has reached a point of hysterical tears, it is important to calm them down before attempting to satisfy their hunger. A little time spent cuddling, rocking, and crooning should calm him just enough.

SAVE YOUR TEARS

Newborn babies are actually incapable of producing tears until they are three or four weeks old. Some don't develop this trait until four or five months of age. Human beings are the only mammals that are known to shed tears at times of emotional stress.

30

"TOO MUCH!"

Overstimulation in new babies does not mean the same thing as in older children. Older children suffer from overstimulation when confronted with too many new people or places, or when playing for too long and becoming overly excited. Babies experience more of a "sensory pain" when overstimulated. Too much bright light or loud noise will cause a smaller baby distress and pain, and this frequently leads to tears. At times such as this, the baby needs to be taken to a quiet, darker room and held close. The removal of the stimuli coupled with the soothing presence of a parent should put a stop to the crying.

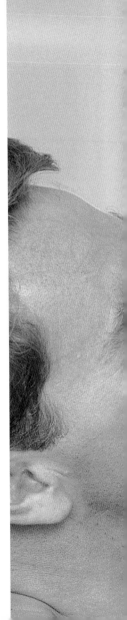

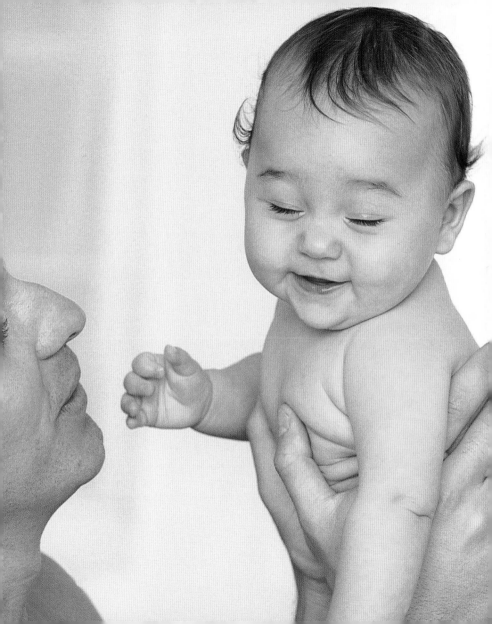

31 "GIVE IT A REST; I'M TRYING TO CHILL."

Surprisingly, infants need time for themselves. When a baby is overstimulated, whether by too much noise and light, or even being passed around from adoring relative to adoring relative, he will need time to calm himself. If he begins to look away from people and show signs of discomfort, perhaps it is time to settle him down in his crib for a few minutes to relax.

TOP BABY NAMES IN 1960

GIRLS	BOYS
1. Lisa	1. Michael
2. Mary	2. David
3. Susan	3. John
4. Karen	4. James
5. Kimberly	5. Robert

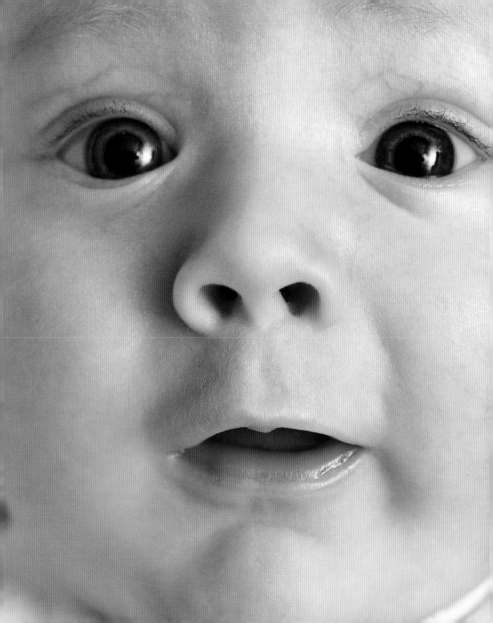

32

"GOTTA PULL IT! GOTTA TOUCH IT!"

When a child reaches the age of around six months, understimulation begins to become a problem. The baby's sensory development is increasing and its brain is crying out for information. When a child's environment offers little or no mental stimulation, this will cause extreme boredom. Boredom leads to tears. The way around this is to make sure it has lots of things to look at, touch, and taste. Toys are great for children of this age, and playthings such as baby gyms and mobiles, offer a complete sensory experience, with buttons, music, and lights.

YOU'RE THE REAL DEAL

Remember that you are your child's first playmate. There is no toy or mobile in the world that is as exciting as you are to your child.

33

"IF AT FIRST YOU DON'T SUCCEED . . ."

As a child grows, she will begin to set herself small yet, to her, extremely important goals. It may be something as simple as throwing a ball, standing, or building a tower of blocks, and inevitably the first failed attempts will be met with frustration and angry tears. The tears are her way of calling the attention of her parents, and with it, some assistance. It can be tempting to step in and do everything for her, just to stop the tears. Instead try to help her complete her goal. If she is trying to reach something a little too high, lift her up so she can grab it herself. If she wants to build a tower, do it together and praise her efforts. That way she will get an enormous sense of achievement and will feel like she can do anything if she keeps trying.

34 "CHILL."

When attempting to calm a crying baby, it is important
to remember that infants can be well-tuned into the body
language of others. Although it is upsetting when dealing
with a child who won't stop crying, it is important not to let
your body language reflect your frustrations. It is easy to
make sharp or erratic movements when agitated or tense, and
this will make your baby insecure and amplify her fears even
further. You may not feel like it, but try to make your body
language relaxed and calm. This will have an amazing effect
on your child.

FEEL THE HEAT

Young babies cannot control their body temperatures in the same way adults
can. The sweat glands in an infant are not fully developed and they lack
the motor skills to remove any blankets or clothes. The one thing they can
do if they become overheated is cry. Unfortunately, the act of crying will
push a baby's temperature up even further. Always monitor your newborn's
temperature, never allowing him to get too hot or too cold.

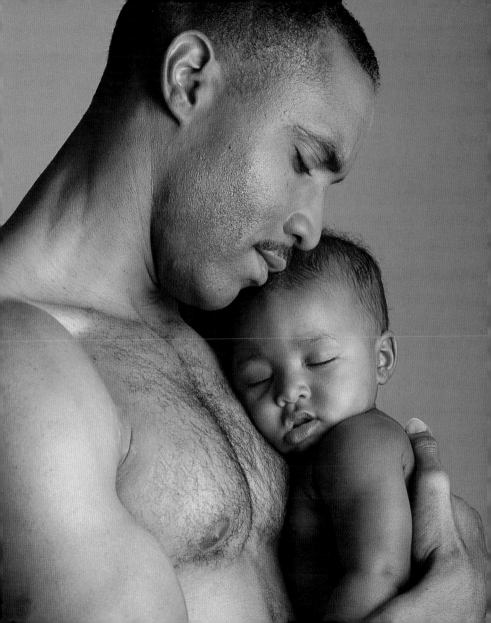

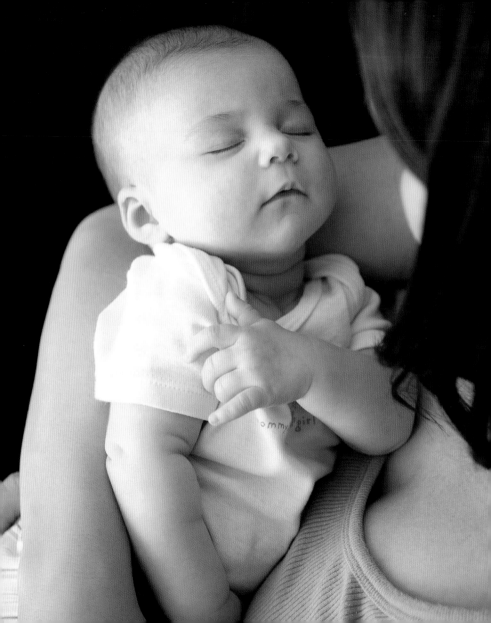

35 "ROCK-A-BYE BABY."

When a child is newly born, one of the most effective ways of soothing them is to rock them backward and forward. Should your older child become upset and in need of consolation, you may find yourself with a distressed toddler on your lap who is trying to rock you instead of the other way around. Such behavior is their subtle way of telling you they need calming and wish to feel the security they felt when rocked in your arms as a smaller child.

HEARTBEAT

Most mothers when rocking their infants will automatically slow to a pace of sixty to seventy rocks per minute, with each movement no more than a few inches. It has been suggested that such movement reminds the baby of their time in the womb, buffeted about by the movements of their mother. However, most people do not move so slowly and it is more likely that such measured pace reflects the sounds of his mother's heartbeat—at around seventy-two beats per minute.

36 "I'LL GET THE HANG OF IT SOONER OR LATER."

It is always exciting for parents to introduce their children to new experiences. When babies become old enough to eat solid food it is often a very messy affair with more food going around the baby's mouth than in it. One of the most helpful things a parent can do, and often does instinctively, is mimic the action of chewing and swallowing for their child. For months now your child has been learning from your example and there are few more effective ways to communicate than by demonstration. Be patient, clean up the mess, and keep showing them what to do. They will get there soon.

EXQUISITE TASTE

Babies actually have more taste buds than adults, and they cover every surface inside their mouths, even on the insides of their cheeks. In the early months of life, babies like sweetness. All other flavors are disliked and may even cause distress. As adults, we often revert to this childish preference for sweet foods in times of stress or depression, perhaps subconsciously reminding ourselves of a much simpler time in our lives.

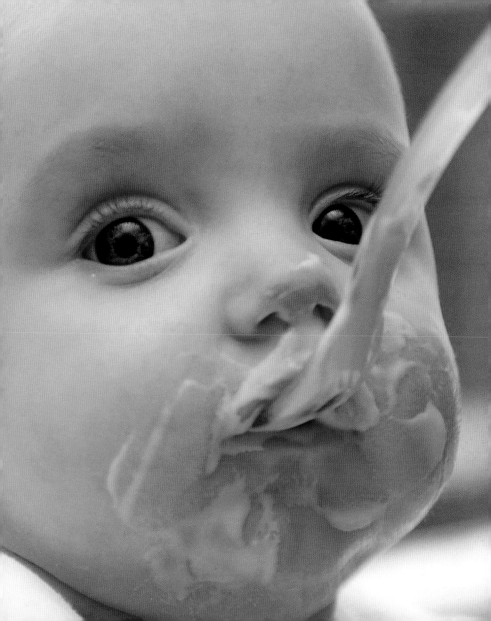

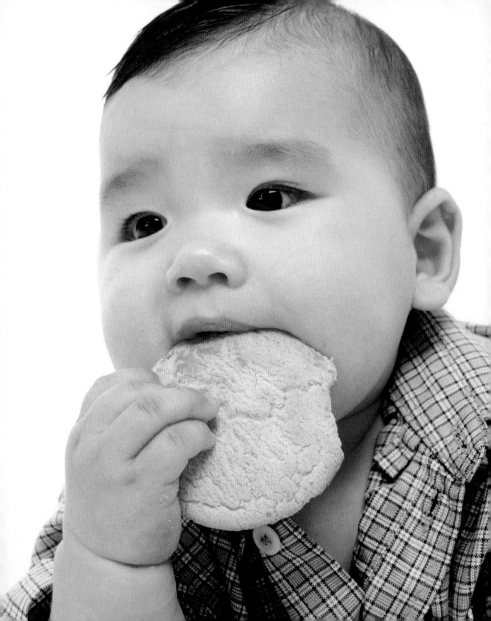

37 "THIS TASTES GREAT. I COULD EAT A LOT OF THESE."

How can you tell when your baby is ready to try solid foods? There are subtle hints. All babies have a "tongue thrust" reflex, which they use to push objects out of their mouths. If they still push out their tongue and gag when you try to spoon-feed them, they may not be ready yet. On the other hand, if they seem distracted while on the bottle or breast, grab at food, and are happy to taste anything, they are ready.

CHEW-CHEW TRAIN

In many tribal cultures, babies are weaned by the mother prechewing food into a slushy mess and then passing it directly into the baby's mouth from hers by pressing her lips together. This action is thought to be the genesis of kissing in our modern culture.

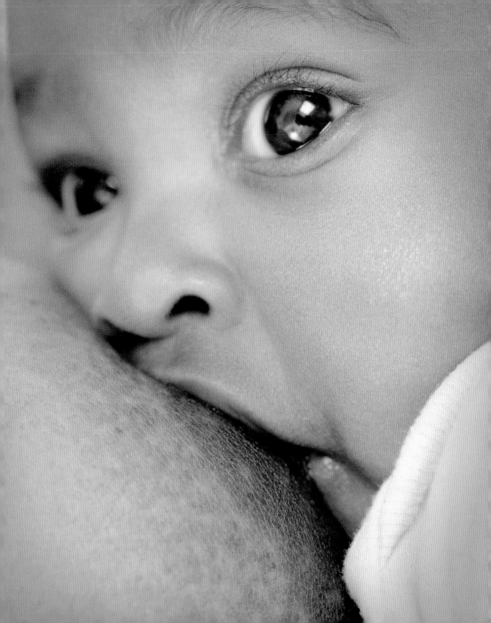

38 "WHERE'S THAT NIPPLE GONE?"

Perhaps one of the most endearing traits of a newborn baby is called "rooting," which is your child's way of letting you know he is hungry. When anything touches his cheek—or, more particularly, his mouth—he will turn his head quickly toward it and try to suckle. Babies, especially newborns, are single-minded in their search for the breast and it often doesn't matter who is cradling them or where they are. Whether cradled on your lap or resting on your shoulder, they will move their heads around trying to find that elusive nipple. If they can't find it, then an ear, a chin, or even a shirt will do!

SWEET

As mentioned previously, babies love the taste of anything sweet. Interestingly, only by stimulating the sweet taste buds will a baby begin to suckle. In fact, when given a number of liquids with increasing levels of sweetness, babies suck harder and longer when the sweet taste is stronger.

39

"THIS IS MY FAVORITE PART OF THE DAY."

For the first few weeks after birth, you may notice that your baby usually closes her eyes when feeding. She isn't sleepy, she is just concentrating completely on the taste sensations. By cutting out all visual stimuli, she can immerse herself in the joy of feeding. When she reaches three months old she may alternate between sucking and looking intently at her mother. Soon after this she will stare intently while feeding, and this mutual gazing strengthens the bond between mother and baby.

NOT ONLY SHEEP . . .

Mothers also have the amazing ability to recognize their baby purely by smell. If mother and baby remain in contact with each other during that important first hour after birth, when tested six hours later the mother will be able to pick out her baby solely by smell.

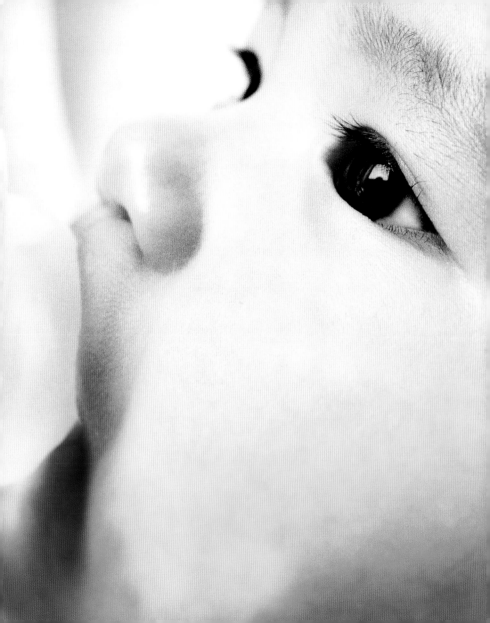

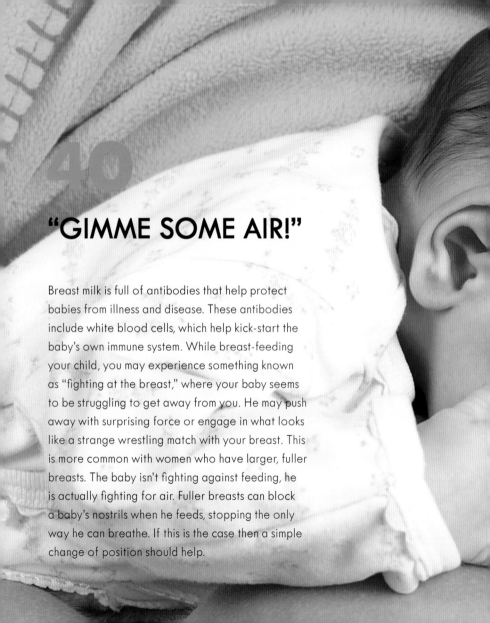

40

"GIMME SOME AIR!"

Breast milk is full of antibodies that help protect babies from illness and disease. These antibodies include white blood cells, which help kick-start the baby's own immune system. While breast-feeding your child, you may experience something known as "fighting at the breast," where your baby seems to be struggling to get away from you. He may push away with surprising force or engage in what looks like a strange wrestling match with your breast. This is more common with women who have larger, fuller breasts. The baby isn't fighting against feeding, he is actually fighting for air. Fuller breasts can block a baby's nostrils when he feeds, stopping the only way he can breathe. If this is the case then a simple change of position should help.

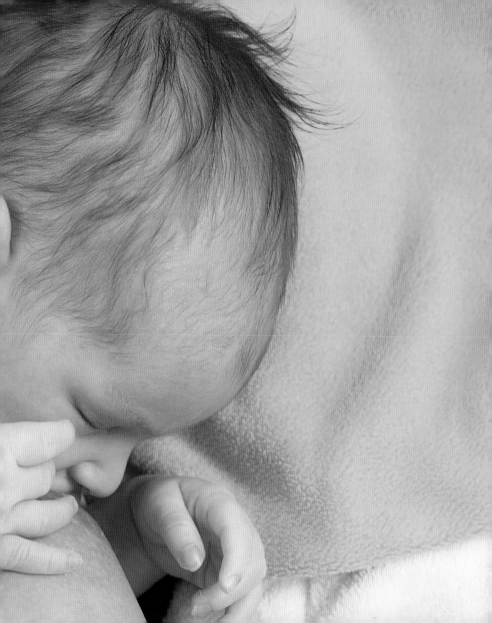

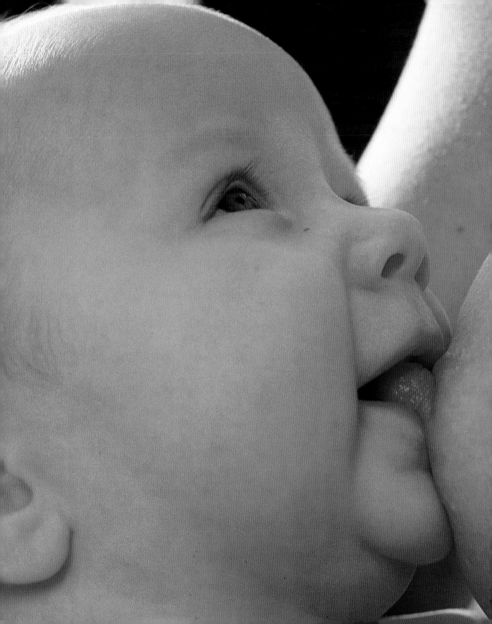

41

"THAT WAS GREAT, BUT I'M STUFFED NOW."

When feeding your child, whether by breast or spoon-feeding, it is sometimes difficult to know whether she has had enough. The common signal that your child will give is turning away from any proffered food. When a young infant has drunk enough milk, she will push out her tongue and turn her head sharply to the side, dislodging the nipple. This shaking of the head and pulling out the tongue has developed into a universal gesture of rejection, even in adult body language.

BREAST IS SLIMMING BEST

Not only is it an important part of the bonding process, but breast-feeding also helps mothers get back into shape after the birth by stimulating weight loss and encouraging the uterus to shrink back to normal size.

42

"YEP, THAT HIT THE SPOT."

Sometimes your infant will show signs of distress just after a feeding. Her legs will kick and her whole body will squirm around as she tries to get comfortable. This is usually the effect of air getting trapped in her stomach and it occurs more regularly in children who are bottle-fed. The way to ease her pain is by keeping her in an upright position as close to the warmth of your body as you can. Rest her on your chest or shoulder and rub her back gently. This will usually help the air escape and it might even send her off to sleep.

WINDED

Should you need to lie your baby down when she is suffering from gas pains, it is much better to rest her on her right-hand side, as this will allow the gas to escape easily.

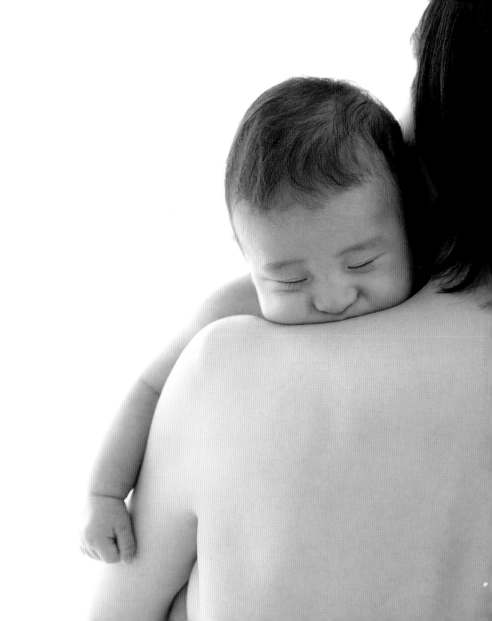

43 "I GET IT, THE FIRST WORD YOU WANT ME TO SAY IS 'MOM,' RIGHT?"

Before learning to talk, your child will experiment with many different sounds. They will try anything from sneezing to coughing or screeching and all of these are a way to get your attention. After a few months they'll begin practicing vowel sounds. It is important to encourage these experiments by joining in. Sit close to your child and emulate the same sounds. Your child will feel rewarded and will soon understand that you are communicating with them, if in a very basic way.

HIGH FIDELITY

A baby's hearing is fully developed by the end of his first month, although he will pay more attention to some sounds than others. High-pitched sounds will grab your child's attention much more than lower-pitched noises. This is why many parents automatically use a higher, squeakier voice when talking to a baby.

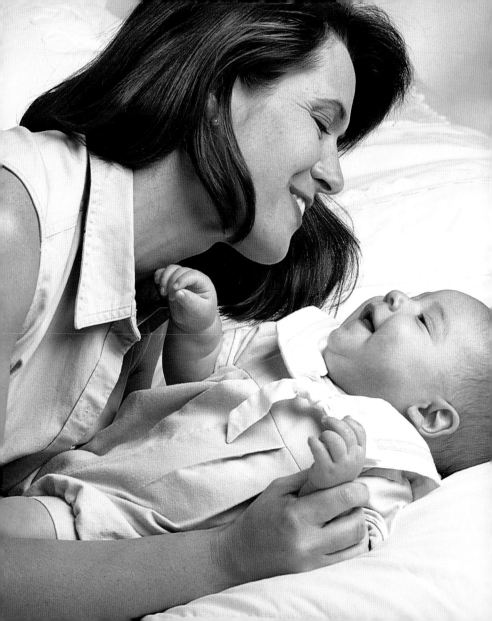

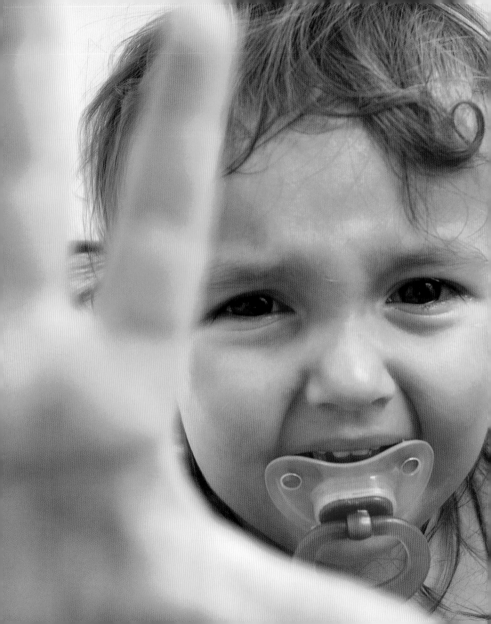

44 "LOOK, I JUST TOLD YOU THAT! DIDN'T YOU HEAR ME GURGLE?"

Learning to speak can be frustrating for toddlers. Often when toddlers try to communicate verbally, they become upset, especially when they feel misunderstood. As a parent, it is important to watch out for the signs that warn when your toddler is about to lose her temper. She may begin to pout, or her body movements could become more emphatic and sharp. If not handled quickly and carefully, you may find yourself with an extremely aggravated child. Redirection is invaluable in these situations. Draw her attention away from the problem and toward something else, such as a favorite book or toy.

LOOK WHO'S TALKING

At twelve to eighteen months old, a young child will begin to recognize the importance of speech and will learn very quickly. She may start by using up to twenty basic words that only she and her parents can understand clearly. For example, she may say "bo bo" for "bottle" while pointing to her bottle. She may hold out her arms and use a word that only you could interpret as "carry."

"SHE REALLY DOESN'T UNDERSTAND. I'LL HAVE TO SKETCH IT."

Toddlers become adept at showing you what they need through body language. After all, she knows you can understand her and she desperately wants to be understood. For example, she will show you when she is tired by rubbing her eyes. She will hand you a book and sit on your lap to show she wants to spend some quality time with you. Encourage this behavior and ask her questions to reinforce the idea you understand what she is, or isn't, saying.

LOOK WHO'S TALKING TWO

By two years old, your child will have mastered 200 words, but will use only fifty of them on a regular basis. On average, a child of this age will add ten more words to her repertoire every day. However, if she is determined to talk, this may increase to one new word every ninety minutes!

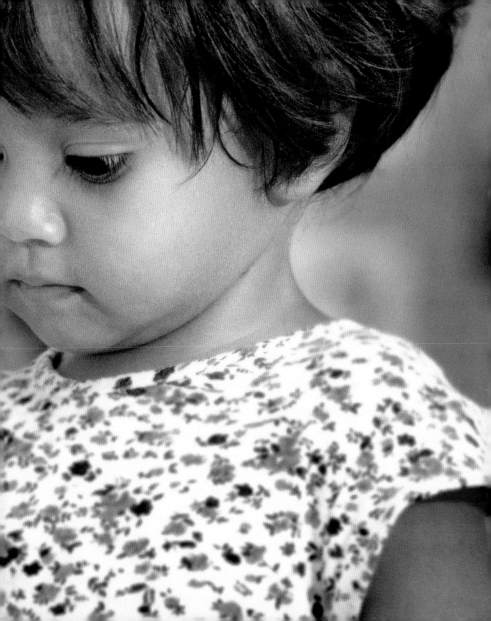

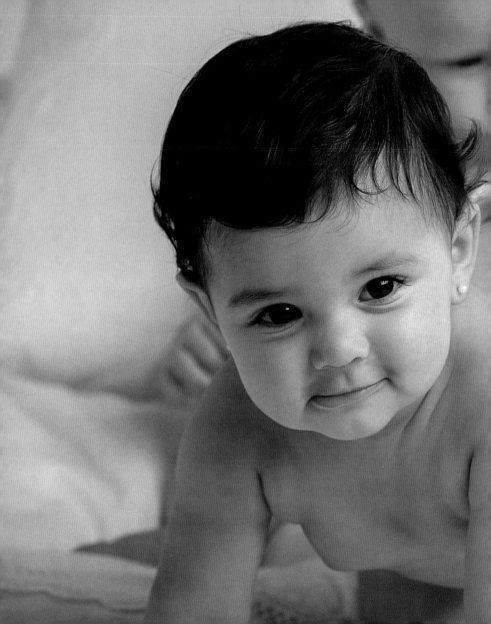

"HERE WE GO. ONE SMALL STEP FOR TODDLERKIND . . ."

As time passes, a child will yearn to do all the things it sees adults doing, including the most challenging of all—walking. This does not happen overnight; a baby goes through several stages before attempting to walk unaided. At the age of three months you will notice that if you stand your baby on a hard surface and support him, he will begin to flex and straighten his knees until, after weeks of practice, he can carry his weight on his legs and will often bounce in excitement.

LOOK WHO'S WALKING

There are many useful items available that encourage the strengthening of the knee and leg muscles. Baby walkers and bouncers are ideal and also a lot of fun.

47

"PHASE ONE, MISSION ACCOMPLISHED. WE HAVE LIFTOFF."

The next stage of learning to walk, known as "cruising," appears between six and nine months. Your baby will begin to pull herself up into a standing position and walk sideways while clinging onto the furniture. This is normally a time of bumps and bruises as your child struggles to maneuver around the room on unsteady legs. Despite the difficulties, there is a steadfast determination and soon, with much practice, your child will become adept at exploring the room via each piece of furniture.

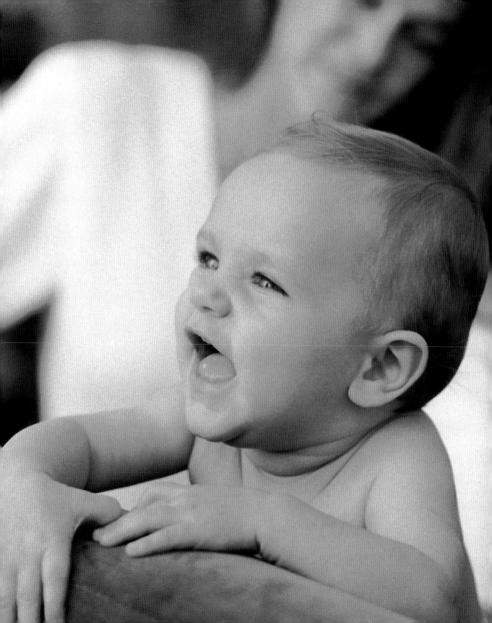

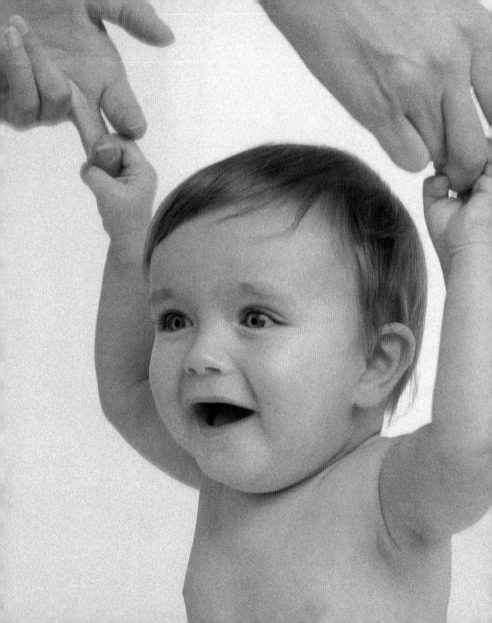

48

"WOW, THIS IS THE REAL THING!"

Between nine and twelve months your baby will be ready to begin walking with adult help. She will demonstrate her eagerness by tightly gripping both of your outstretched hands and leading you around. This is an exciting time for both child and parent as unaided walking is not far away. It may also be a little backbreaking for mothers and fathers. Holding on to her tiny hands, stooping over slightly so as not to pull her arms, and sometimes carrying her weight if she stumbles can put a strain on adult back muscles, especially if she wants to practice all day long. It is all worth it for the look of sheer joy on her face when she completes her first solo walk.

DON'T PLOW WITH THEM, THOUGH

Pound for pound, babies and toddlers are stronger than oxen, particularly in their legs.

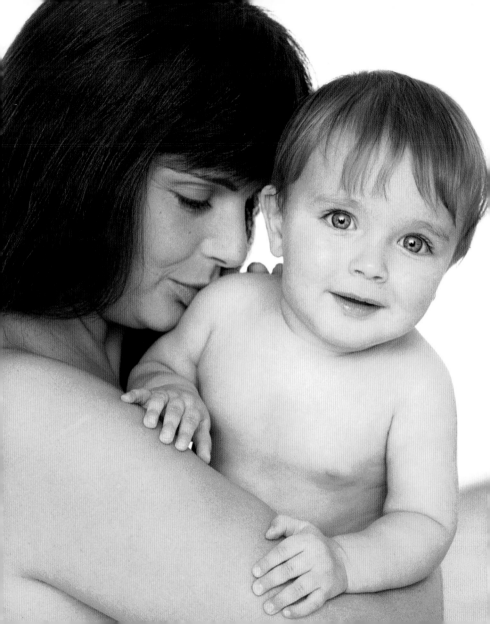

49 "MAYBE I'LL STILL LET MOM CARRY ME TO THE KITCHEN."

As your child learns to walk (at anywhere between ten and eighteen months) you may notice that they become more exploratory. The world is an exciting place. However, the world is also a very scary place. This is why they will run back to the safety of your arms. This behavior can become tiring as a parent, watching your child wander off happily only to come racing back to you, demanding to be picked up. No sooner have you picked them up, than they wriggle and want to be put down again. This is your toddler's way of sampling a little independence while keeping in contact with the most important person in their life. They will come back for reassurance, and once comforted are happy to explore for a little while longer.

QUICK STEP

Amazingly, the average toddler takes 176 steps per minute. It is no wonder chasing after a young child can be exhausting.

50 "NO? SERIOUSLY?"

When studying a child's body language, it is important to pay attention to your own, because he will learn from you. As your child grows, he may begin to display behavior you disapprove of. This is when disciplinary signals from you become important. Basic signs of "disapproval" include frowning, shaking your head, and a firm tone of voice. All of these send the powerful message that you do not agree with what he has done. This can be upsetting for a child as he looks for your approval every day. Studies suggest that if used early enough in your child's development, then later on a simple frown or shake of the head will be enough to chastise him when he has been naughty.

VERY, VERY BAD

If you discover your child doing something very wrong then you can use much stronger negative body language. For example, a louder voice, quick movements, and a cast-iron glare are effective. Although these are more forceful, stern signals, it is important not to become physically aggressive. Should you feel that way, it is best to leave the room until you calm down.

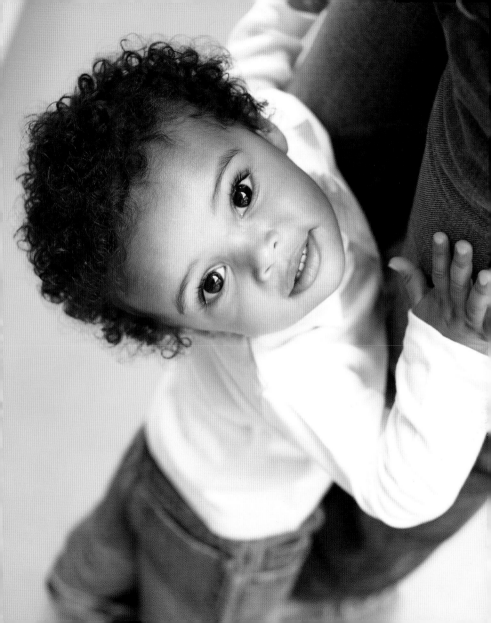

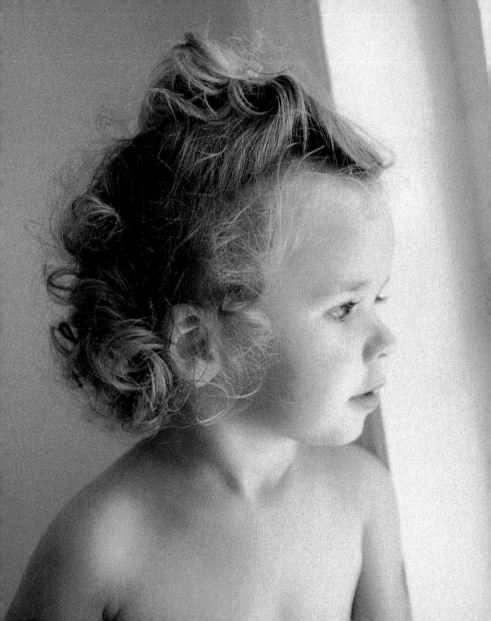

51 "I AM LISTENING, REALLY."

When your child becomes older and able to better communicate verbally as well as physically, you may notice that when you talk to her she may appear not to listen. She may not look at you, continue playing, or simply not acknowledge that you have said anything. She has yet to learn that it is polite to look people in the eye when they talk, or to nod in agreement. It is not that she can't hear you, but that she doesn't yet know how to use these necessary nonverbal signals. Here, it is important for you to provide a good example with your own body language. When you speak, physically get down to her level so you can look her in the eyes. If she is distracted, simply touch her to gain her attention. Ask her if she has understood and teach her to nod if she has.

DON'T SHOUT

It can be frustrating if you feel your child is ignoring you and you may be tempted to make yourself louder by shouting. Unfortunately, this causes your child to ignore you even more, as she becomes immune to your shouts. One gentle touch on the face will have more power than a dozen loud words.

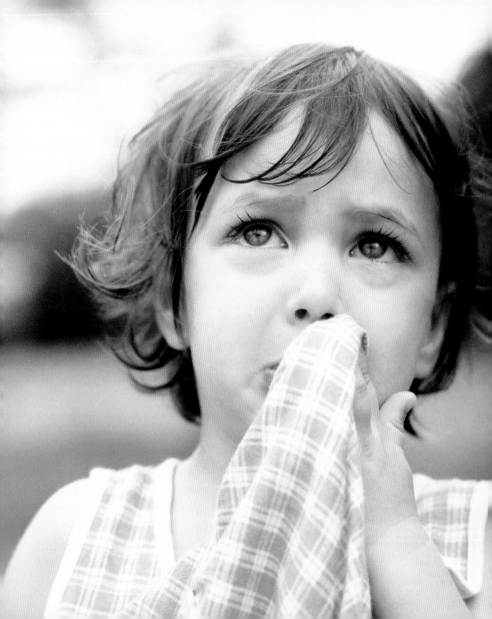

52 "SORRRRY."

As your child develops, you will find it increasingly necessary to chastise her for bad behavior. Around the two-year mark a child will begin to test the boundaries you have laid down for her, and sometimes you will need to stand your ground and scold her. But how can you tell if your child is truly sorry for her bad behavior? Once again, her body language will reflect her real attitude. When she is truly sorry, she will display some universal appeasement signals. She may bow her head while listening to you—a widely used signal of obedience in the animal kingdom. Anyone who has chastised a dog will have witnessed the same behavior. She will also want to be close to you, hugging and touching or even hanging off her mother's clothes, just like baby chimps cling to the fur of their mothers.

ACCENTUATE THE POSITIVE

Babies will repeat actions that elicit positive responses from their parents. For example when a baby smiles, her parents will smile and praise her for her actions, thus encouraging her to do it again. Disciplining your child should also be done in a positive manner. Instead of reserving comment for any naughty behavior, make sure you praise and reward all the good behavior. This will encourage your child to be well-behaved.

53 "NOT REALLY SORRY."

If after chastising your child you suspect she is not really sorry for her behavior, there are certain body language signals that can help. Watch for signs that your child is not taking her apology seriously. Gritted teeth, a strained, unnatural voice, or perhaps clenched fists all point to a child apologizing purely because she feels she has to, and not from any real remorse. She may also suppress a smile or smirk if she feels as though she has tricked you into accepting her apology. She may become tense when you try to hug her and be resistant to any affection. All these signs point to unresolved aggression that the insincere apology has not dispersed.

"SORRY" SHOULDN'T BE THE HARDEST WORD

Make sure you are providing a good example when you apologize. Many adults make the mistake of saying they are sorry to a child in a dismissive manner, as if the feelings of the child are not really significant. This sends the message that apologies are not important and do not have to be heartfelt. Maintain eye contact, and speak in an even, serious tone. When they see how sorry you are they will realize how good it feels when someone respects their feelings in this way.

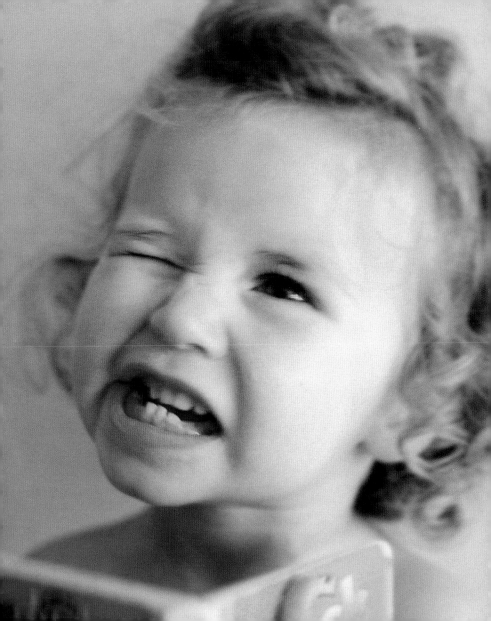

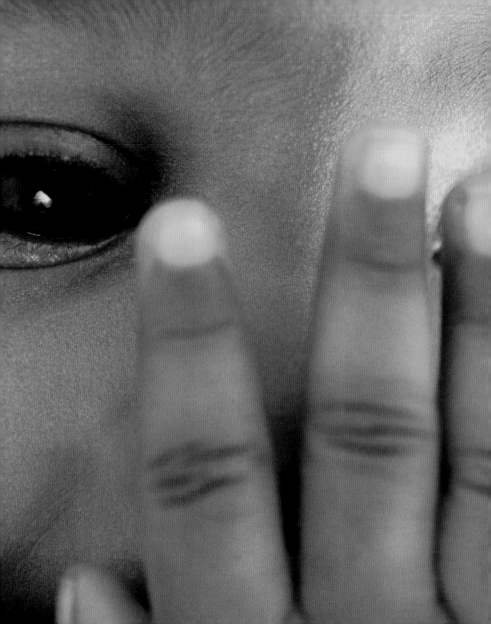

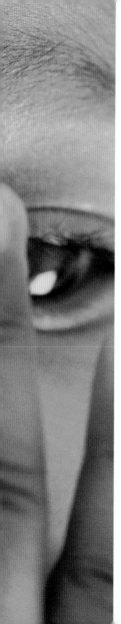

54

"IT'S TRUE, THE GLASS JUMPED OFF THE TABLE ALL BY ITSELF."

As children develop, their language skills and words slowly evolve into comprehensible sentences. Another milestone soon occurs—your child's first attempt at lying. Fortunately for the parents, body language will certainly reveal the truth. When a child first tries to lie to his parents, he will not maintain steady eye contact, or he may cover his mouth with his hand, or he might hang his head and look at the floor. His body language will give signs of nervousness that would be unwarranted if he were telling the truth.

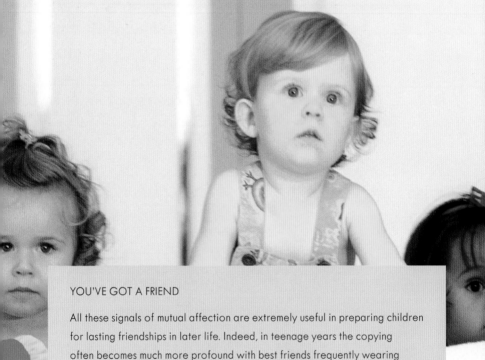

55 "LET'S HAVE A GIRLS' NIGHT EVERY NIGHT!"

YOU'VE GOT A FRIEND

All these signals of mutual affection are extremely useful in preparing children for lasting friendships in later life. Indeed, in teenage years the copying often becomes much more profound with best friends frequently wearing the same clothes and listening to the same music. It is a natural expression of "togetherness."

As your child grows, she will come into contact with more children her own age. When children take delight in each other's company there are some very definite signals they send out. They will become excited with lots of jumping up and down and noisemaking. They will also find reasons to touch, whether it is through a welcoming hug or just a more restrained touch of hands. These are all signs that your child is comfortable with her friend and enjoys her company. As they get older you will see them copying each other's actions. This matching of body language is an important bonding process and even extends to the rate at which they breathe.

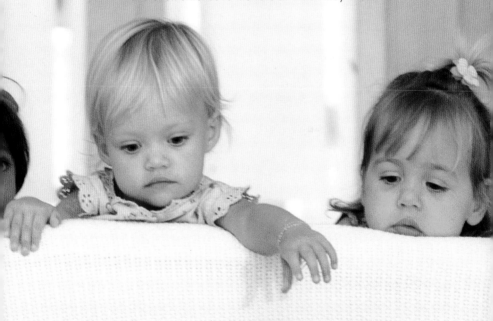

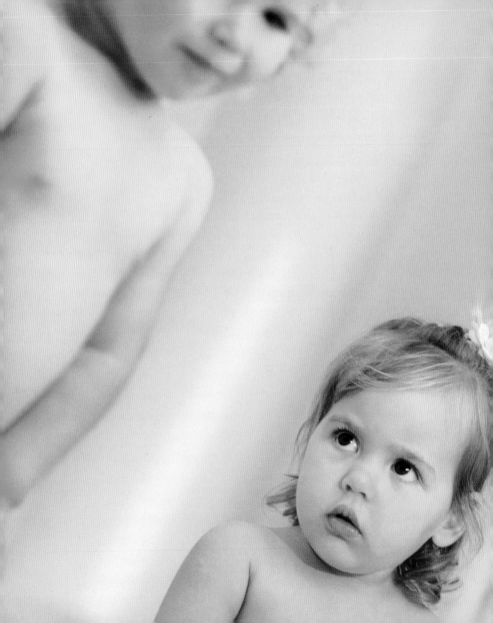

56 "SHE STOLE THE BALL. SHE DID! SHE DID!"

Just as there are signals to show if your child likes her new playmate, there are also signs to show whether she doesn't. If unhappy or unsure in the presence of another child, she will not attempt to touch or welcome her friend. Neither will she try to match her body language and may become much more focused on you, sometimes becoming clingy and even aggressive toward the "interloper." In older children there will be more outward signals of dislike such as mockery. If you notice behavior such as this it is important not to try and force the friendship. Your child will make friends eventually, but of their own choosing.

BLUE FOR A BOY?

The tradition of dressing boys in blue stems from ancient times when superstition was rife. Boy children were—at that time—valued more than girls. Also many people feared the influence of evil spirits or demons on their children. To protect their male offspring, they dressed them in a color considered holy or lucky: blue.

57 "I'M FINE ALL BY MYSELF."

If you are concerned that your child doesn't seem to want to make friends and spends too much time on her own, do not worry. First take a look at her body language. Some children become sensitive around too many people and prefer the company of one or two individuals. Being surrounded by lots of people can make them nervous. Watch her actions when she is faced with a group of children. If she turns away from them, plays happily on her own, appears not to notice them at all, and will neither match her body language to theirs nor look up from her game, she is happy in her own little world— and is not lonely.

SPOTTING AUTISM

There has been much in the media about children with autism and how to spot the telltale signals that all is not well with your child. Autistic children have trouble playing pretend games, don't show interest in objects pointed out to them, find disruption of routine extremely difficult, and avoid eye contact or touch or playing with other children. Should you have real fears, it is always best to speak to your doctor.

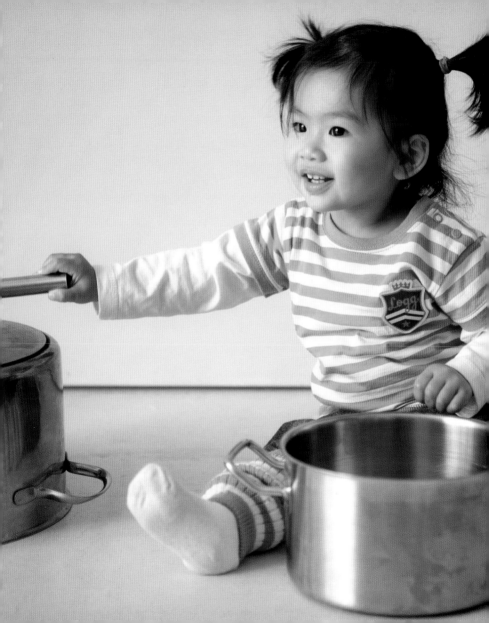

58

"NOT GOING TO JOIN IN."

A lonely child will exhibit different behavior from a child who is happy on her own. She will turn to face other children in a group, studying them from a distance. She will match her body language to theirs and find it difficult to concentrate on anything else. Her movements will become tentative and she may look very unhappy. It is your job to instruct her in the skills of forming a relationship with other children. Perhaps you should take her hand and help her to introduce herself to the others, ask them what game they are playing, and ask whether they mind another child joining in.

CONFIDENCE BOOSTER

If your older child is feeling lonely or excluded, trying to fix the situation for her may not be the best solution. Not all children pick up social skills easily. Encourage her not to give up and let her talk openly about her feelings. The best thing you can do as a parent is boost her confidence so she feels able to make her own friends.

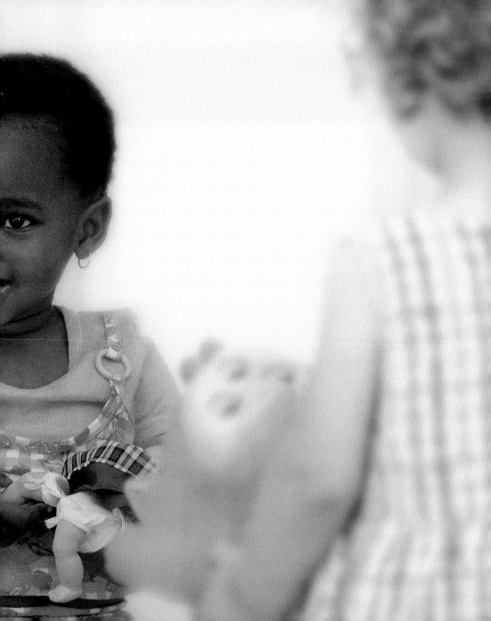

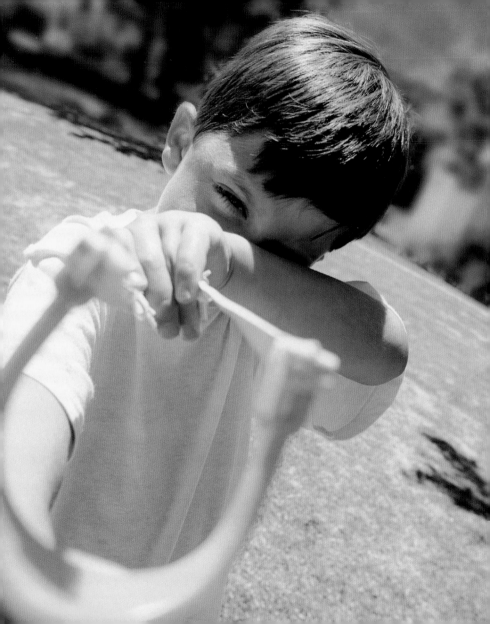

59 "OLDER KIDS ARE WAY TOO SCARY."

Unfortunately, many young children will run into others who are actively aggressive toward them and this will often cause them to become more introverted or even fearful. The signs that your child is being bullied are often very subtle as no one, not even a young child, likes to admit they are being victimized. Watch out for unexpected or unwarranted crying, mood swings, loss of appetite, and lack of sleep. This is an opportunity to teach your child how to use body language effectively. Bullies of any age will pick on easy targets; they don't want trouble. Teach your child to tell them firmly and loudly to leave them alone and then walk away.

60

"I WANT TO MEET EVERYBODY."

Every parent wants their child to be confident and outgoing, but how can you tell if they really are? The answer is to watch her movements when faced with a group of peers, or even adults. A confident child will have a steady posture, she will look people in the eye and her movements will be measured and composed. In her eyes, there will be no question that she will be liked and accepted—of course she will!

BLUE EYES

Babies' eyes are almost always blue when first born, though most will slowly darken and turn brown by the age of six months. Should the irises remain clear and blue at six months, the child will have blue eyes.

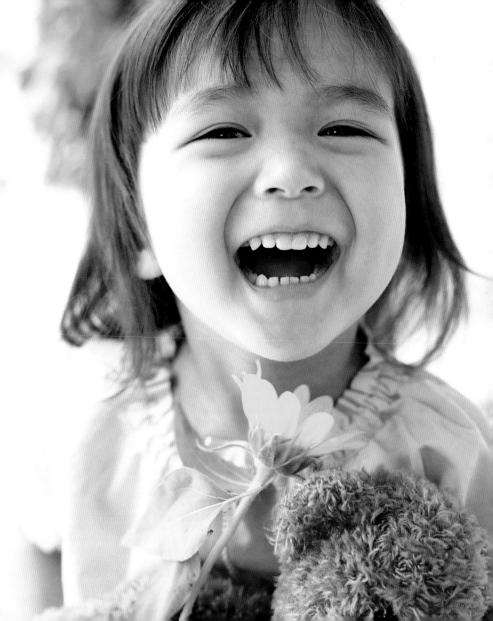

61

"I WANT THEM TO GO AWAY."

A child who is not confident will display completely different gestures from the ones discussed in the previous entry. She will be reticent in joining a group and may be hesitant to leave the safety of her mother's arms. Her posture will be uneven, or limp with hunched or raised shoulders—all signs of tension. Worry will be etched on her face and her movements may become uncoordinated or clumsy.

BONDING SKILLS

Children slowly learn how to make friends of their own age by building on the friendship they have with their parents. A child who has bonded well with her mother and father will find it easier to expand her own circle of close friends.

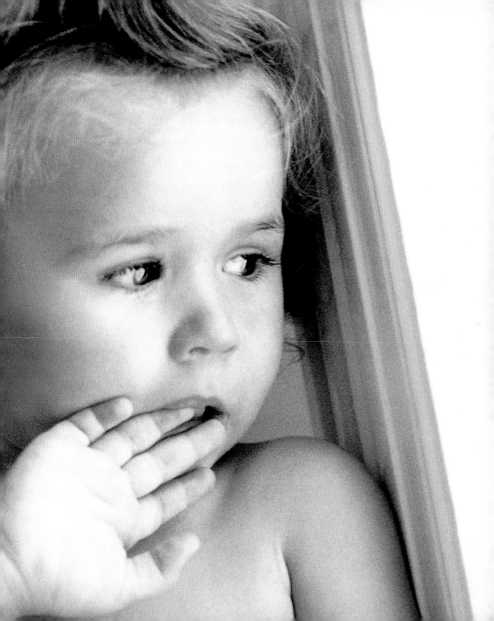

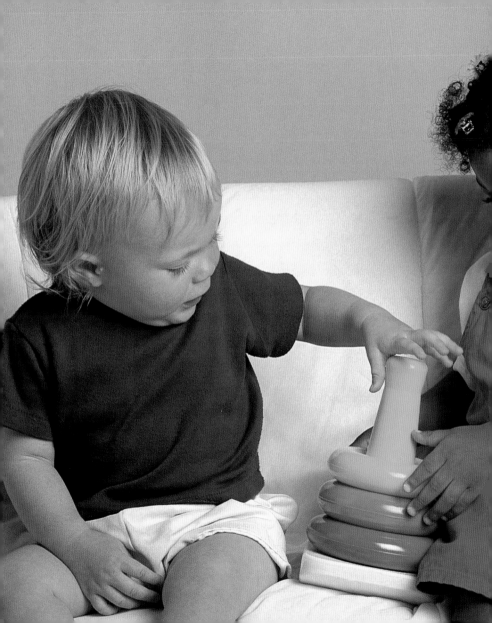

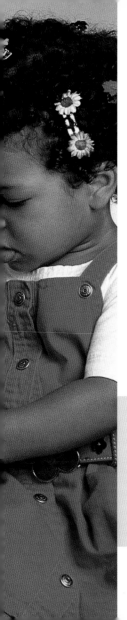

62

"WHERE'S THE RED ONE GONE?"

By his second year, your child will begin to make friends of his own age. It can be a slow process as he may still be quite shy and lacking the skills necessary to form friendships immediately. You may notice him playing alongside others and occasionally joining in, only to go off on his own again. Relax and don't push him. He is just getting used to how the whole thing works and may not yet have grasped the idea of sharing. Be patient. He will get there.

PARALLEL PLAY

"Parallel play" is a normal stage in the child's development and is a toddler's way of getting comfortable with his playmate. He will play side by side, engaged in different activities, but occasionally stop and watch what his neighbor is doing.

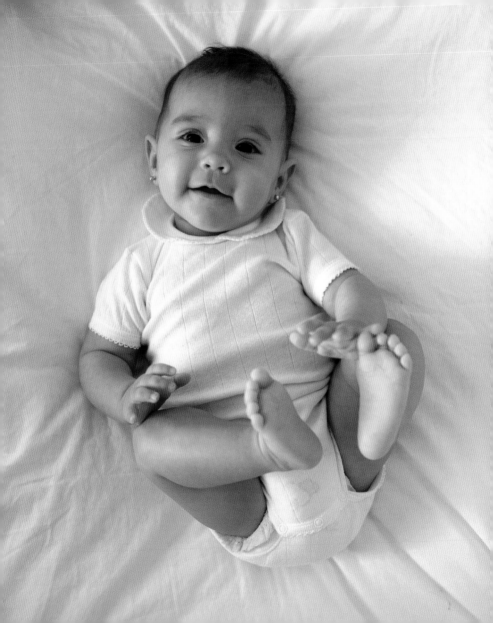

63 "IT'S ONLY ROCK 'N' ROLL, BUT I LIKE IT."

From around nine months of age, some babies begin to rock themselves for long periods of time. They will sit and swing their bodies back and forth; sometimes they will lie in bed and try and rock themselves to sleep. This self-rocking points to a child in severe need of more affection and physical closeness with their parents. Prolonged bouts of self-rocking should be interpreted as a sign of distress and unhappiness. Try holding your child gently as he rocks, do your best to calm him with soft words or singing, and try to sway him gently instead of allowing him to rock himself. All these actions can help him feel more secure and slowly cancel out the need for self-rocking.

DON'T STOP THE ROCK

Self-rocking usually begins at around six months and stops before your child reaches his third birthday. Many children will use self-rocking sporadically, for example as a distraction when experiencing physical pain. Some children rock themselves when simply singing or humming a tune.

64 "LET'S GET NAKED. NAKED IS FUN!"

Around two years of age, you may notice some strange and often embarrassing habits in your child. One of the most mortifying is a toddler's tendency to shed his clothes. This is all well and good if you are at home, but what if it happens in the supermarket or at a friend's house? Usually this kind of exhibitionist behavior is triggered by boredom and this is your child's way of telling you his feelings. It is a fairly extreme form of body language, but one that will often do the trick. It certainly grabs your attention!

BEATING THE BOREDOM

If you find yourself in this situation, the best thing to do is involve your child in what you are doing. If you are grocery shopping, set him a task. If you are in the fruit aisle, ask him if he can point to or find the bananas. Keep the game going as long as you need to finish your shopping.

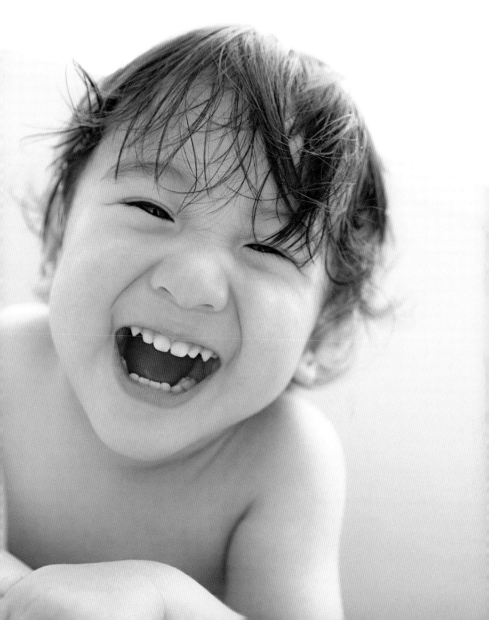

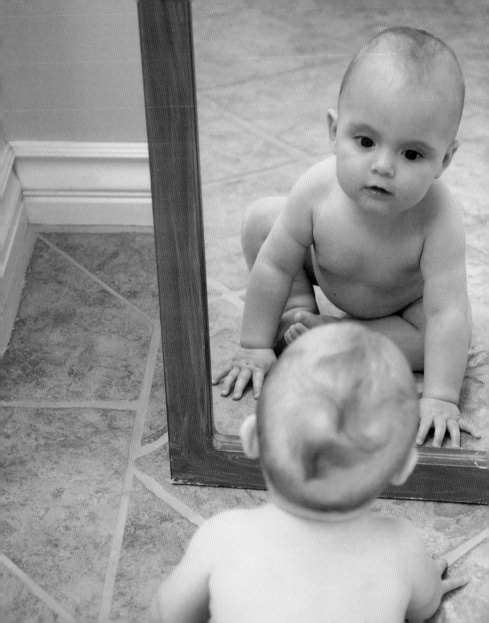

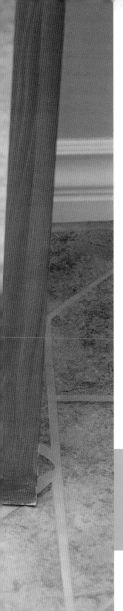

65

"THEY'RE INTERESTING."

During the first year of childhood, babies often become fascinated by their own reflections, kissing and stroking the baby they see in the mirror. It is delightful to watch as they observe every move the captivating creature in front of them makes, but this is also an important time in the psychological development of a child. According to psychoanalyst Jacques Lacan, the baby believes the mirror image of itself is really its true self. The realization that it is not helps the baby grasp the notion of others and otherness.

"A toddler believes that if you truly love a person, you stay with that person 100 percent of the time."

Lawrence Balter

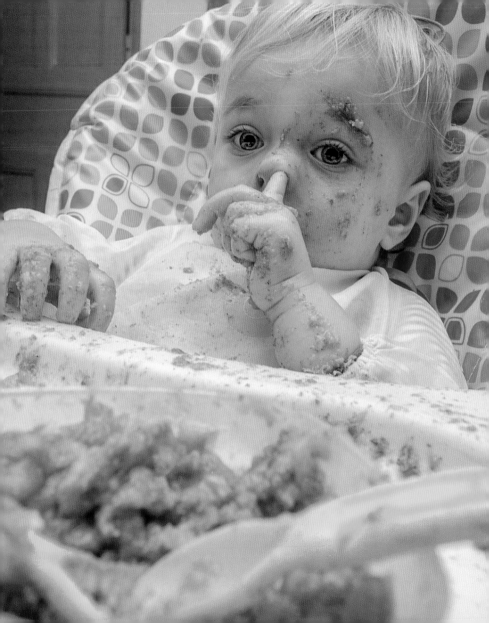

66 "I CAN STUFF IT AAAAAAALLLLLLLLLL THE WAY UP!"

It is a familiar and all too regular sight—your child has his finger lodged firmly up his nose once again. Children are fascinated with their bodies and bodily functions. At this age they are completely uninhibited and they will explore their body the only way they know how—through touch. Not only the nose gets this special attention; any interesting nooks and crevices will be investigated thoroughly or displayed publicly! As a parent the best thing to do in these situations is to teach your child the important difference between "public behavior" and "private behavior." But don't be overly harsh. It would be a shame to force inhibitions onto them at such an innocent age.

NO NOSE IS GOOD NEWS

A good tactic in stopping constant nose picking is to watch your child carefully, and when his hand starts heading for his nose, pass him a tissue and suggest he blows his nose. Don't be angry or appalled; stay calm and don't turn it into a larger issue than it is

67 "WILL YOU JUST LISTEN TO ME?"

Toddlers often display behavior that is undesirable, usually stemming from frustration. Biting is one of the more extreme ways your child may vent his irritations. Just as biting down on something when they were babies relieves the pain of teething, biting on something in later years also relieves more emotional stress. Toddlers tend to bite when feeling helpless, when not getting their own way, or sometimes in self-defense when playtime with other children has turned sour. Occasionally, it is used as a way to get your attention.

THE NAUGHTY STEP

The best way to deal with such aggressive behavior is to deny him the attention he so badly craves. Take him away from all the action, perhaps to his room or a "naughty chair," and leave him there for a couple of minutes. Talk to him firmly and tell him why such behavior will not be tolerated.

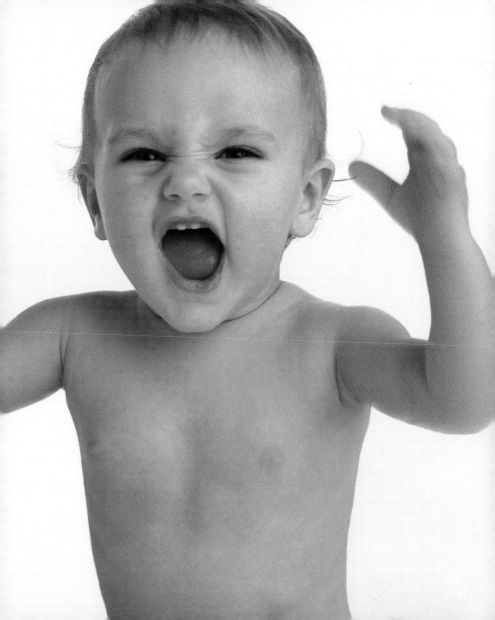

68 "I ONLY DO STRAWBERRY JELLY."

Just after their second birthday, your child, who was once excited by food, may become an extremely picky eater. They will eat much less than they used to and will often refuse anything different or new. Do not panic. Many children at this age experience "neophobia" or a fear of anything new. Their carefully structured routine gives them security and confidence. Even the slightest deviation from what they consider the norm will cause them to be upset and even spark a tantrum—this includes their daily eating habits.

DON'T PANDER TO MISS PICKY

Studies have shown that a picky child needs to be given a new food between fifteen and twenty times before she will even try it. Patience—as always—is key.

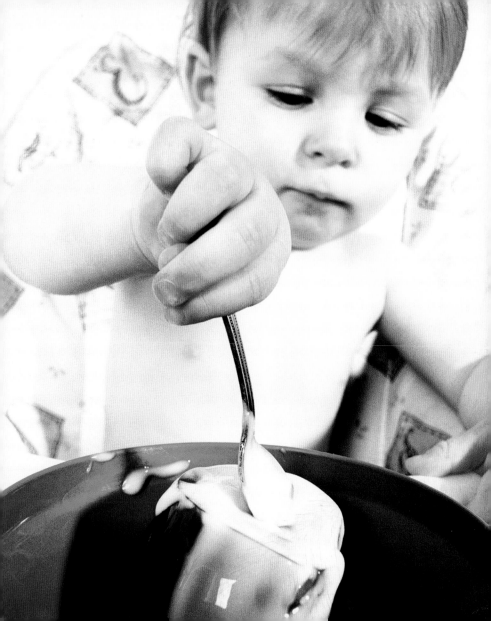

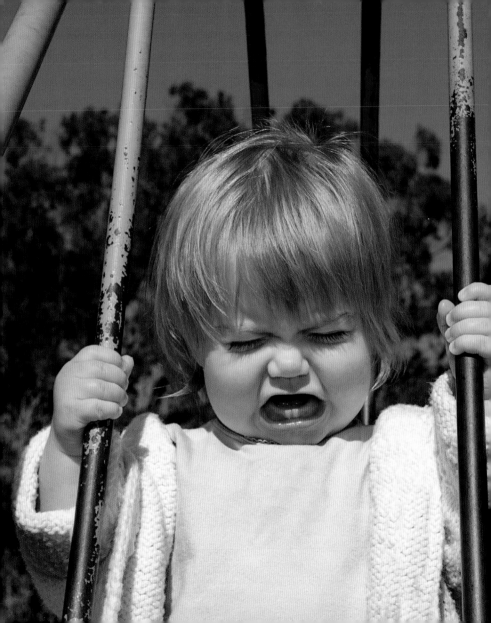

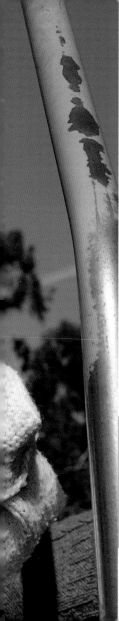

69

"LOOK AT ME NOW!"

Many parents have experienced the worrying habit some children have of banging their heads. When grumpy, upset, or in the middle of a full-blown tantrum, many children will begin to bang their heads against furniture, floors, or even walls. They seem to have no idea of how much they could be hurting themselves, and often this behavior will go on for many minutes. This is usually an attention-seeking device and the child will not do himself any damage. Sometimes, if he is in pain, he will bang his head as a form of distraction. Some children even use it as a way to relieve tension before bedtime.

OUTGROWING THE PHASE

Twenty percent of children will bang their head at one stage or another. It typically appears from six months of age and will stop before the fourth birthday. Boys are four times more likely to do it than girls.

70 "YOU CAN'T BEAT A GOOD THUMB."

A young child happily sucking her thumb is a common sight. Babies will often have pacifiers to do the same job, but some children find the thumb much tastier. Many parents become concerned about this behavior as they suspect it is their child's way of expressing inner insecurities through body language. Most of the time, this is not the case. It is advised that children should stop sucking in between four and five years of age, so as not to cause problems with the teeth. However, 85 percent of children have already stopped by this age. Children like to suck on something when they need comfort, such as when tired or bored.

TO SLEEP, PERCHANCE TO SUCK

Studies have shown that children who suck their thumb as a way of getting to sleep will generally fall asleep faster and will sleep through the night much earlier on than children who do not suck their thumbs.

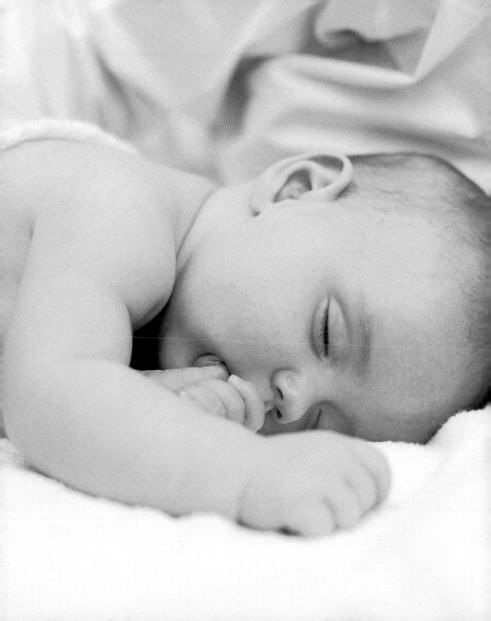

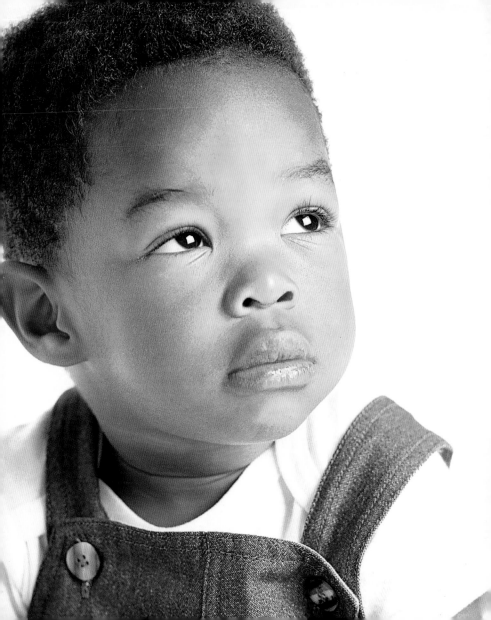

71 "YEAH, TELL ME ABOUT IT."

Children are incredibly sensitive and often understand more than we give them credit for. They listen to every word we say, read our body language, and pick up on our moods. This is why sometimes they also take on our stresses. Childhood stress displays itself in several ways, and if you are feeling under pressure yourself, whether financial, physical, or emotional, make sure your child is not experiencing it, too. Your child may complain of headaches, lack of appetite, have regular nightmares, or become clingy and never want to be alone. Sometimes aggressive or stubborn behavior will appear, or your child may become withdrawn and quiet.

HOME = SAFE

To help relieve the situation, make sure your house is a safe and dependable place. Make sure you take the time to sit and talk to your child about their worries and fears, but never criticize them for having these thoughts.

72

"COME BACK!"

Many babies, when reaching nine months old, will become
clingy and demanding. They will cry every time their mother
leaves the room. They will demand to be held, touched, and
kissed more often than usual. They may even shun their father
as an alternative and will calm down only when safely back in
their mother's arms. This can be very stressful and somewhat
perplexing for both parents. However, it is a normal part of
a child's development called separation anxiety and only
lasts a few months. Right now, the maternal figure is the most
important person in the world and the only one who can make
the world feel safe again.

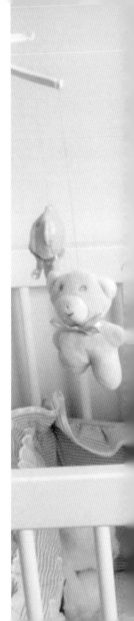

DAD, YOU'RE NEXT

This separation anxiety will commonly switch to the father in
the following months. Soon, Daddy will be the only person
in the world—although this will be for a shorter period.

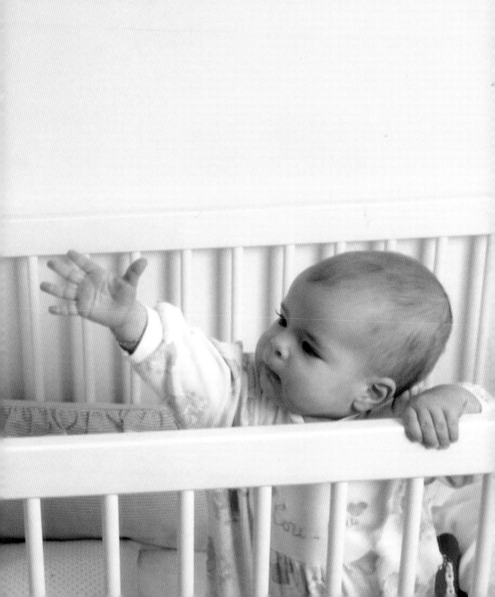

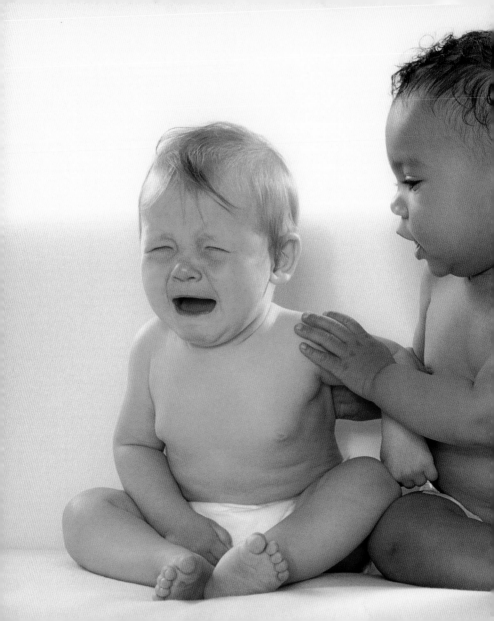

73

"IT'S NOT SO BAD.
YOU'LL BE OKAY."

One of the most frustrating times for a parent is dealing with an unhappy baby. There are few things worse than trying to comfort an inconsolable child. There are some telltale signs that trouble and tears are on the horizon, and if caught in time it is possible to head them off at the pass. If an infant starts to arch his back, distort his face, or attempt to turn away from something, these are clear signals of distress. Try to respond quickly before he becomes too upset. Change his position, cuddle him, or rock him just to let him know you are there.

CRY FREEDOM

Of course this may not always stop the tears. There are times when a baby will cry no matter what. At times like this all you can really do is remain calm and try your best to soothe him until the moment passes.

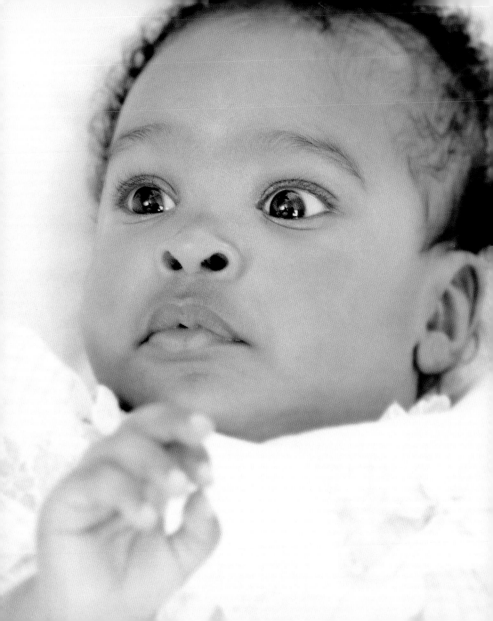

74

"I'M NOT LOOKING AT YOU—GO FIGURE."

Just as in adults, looking at a baby's eyes can give you an enormous amount of information. A happy and content baby will maintain eye contact. On the other hand, if your child avoids meeting your gaze, it may be a sign that she is overexcited and needs some time to calm down and relax. Heavy-lidded or scrunched-up eyes, especially if the baby is frowning, means he is in pain.

JUST A BLUR

A baby's eyes at birth are three-quarters the size of an adult eye. For the following two years, your infant's eyes will continue to develop. Although his eyes are able to see, his brain is not yet ready to process large amounts of information, which is why his eyesight will remain blurred for the first few weeks.

75 "PUT THE ICE CREAM IN THE CART, OR I'LL SCREAM!"

How many times have you sat in a restaurant or gone shopping and seen a child acting out as their helpless parents try anything to calm them down? It's every parent's worst nightmare. The trick is to understand why this happens and notice the signs that indicate when trouble is on the way. Children get excited by crowds—and new things to see, smell, and hear. This speeds the heart rate up. At the same time it is overwhelming being surrounded by so many new sensations. Under the strain, her body literally goes into overload. Watch out for her trying to cut off the stimuli by closing her eyes, huddling inside your coat, or suddenly becoming quiet and still. If this state continues, it will lead to tantrums and tears.

BLOWING OFF STEAM

One of the best remedies for overstimulation is exercise. Take your child outside for a little while and let her run off some of the adrenaline coursing through her system.

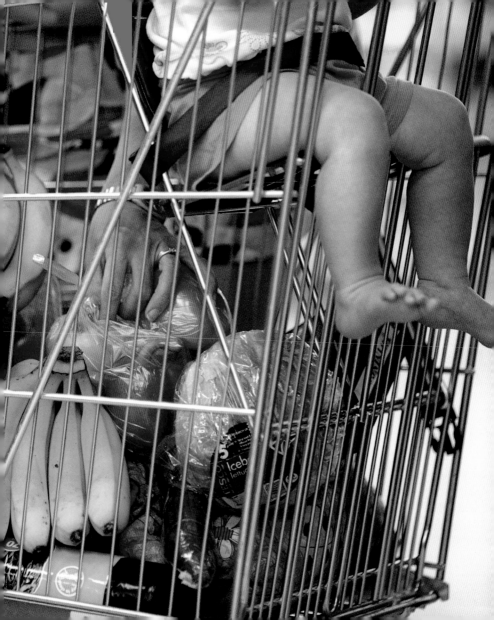

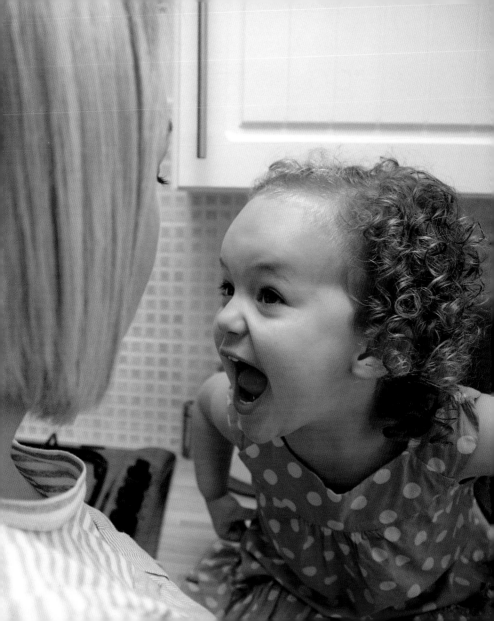

76 "GO ON, ASK ME WHAT YOU'VE DONE WRONG."

It is every parent's dreaded moment: their child's first tantrum. Everyone has seen them—in the grocery store, the toy shop, at nursery school—and we all thank our lucky stars when it isn't our child putting on such a display. Unfortunately, the time will come when it is your child, and how you deal with it will determine how often you will experience tantrums in the future. As he begins to develop his own mind and personality, your child will begin to test the boundaries you have laid down for him. He will want his own way more often and will sometimes use a fit of temper to try and get it. It is important to remain calm and ignore the tantrum—he will eventually run out of steam when he is denied your attention and his way.

NEVER BACK DOWN

The worst thing you can ever do when faced with a childish hissy fit is to back down. By doing this you will reinforce the idea that if he cries enough, he will get his own way.

77

"I'M OKAY, HONEST."

Body language takes all kinds of subtle forms and the rate of breathing is perhaps the most difficult to monitor. Babies take such shallow breaths, especially while asleep, that it's difficult to notice any changes, unless they are dramatic. Usually when a baby is happy or excited, her breathing will quicken. Quite often she will use her entire body to indicate joy; her legs will kick erratically and she may giggle. Should her breathing become faster and deeper at the same time, this often points to trouble ahead. If coupled with a frown or grimace, tears are probably on the way.

NO FRESHENER REQUIRED

Babies' breath smells sweet and fresh compared to adult breath—especially first thing in the morning! The reason for this is the lack of teeth. Bad breath is caused by bacteria that live on the teeth, which rots any trapped food.

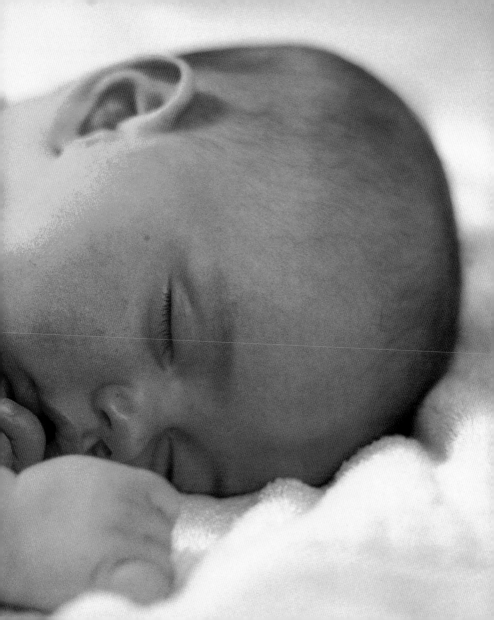

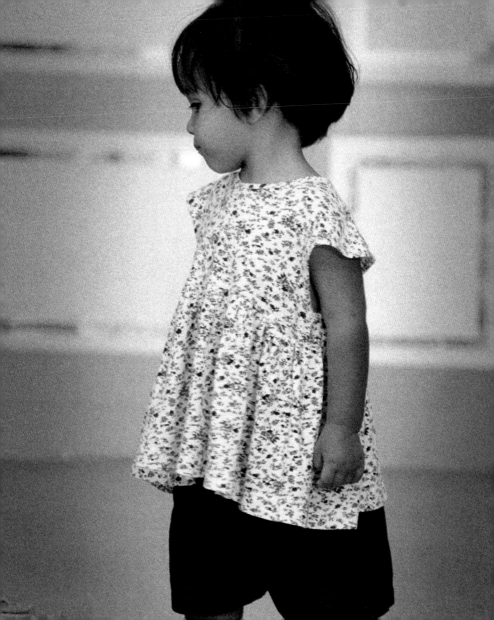

78 "NO, DON'T EVEN THINK ABOUT IT."

One of the most frequently heard words spoken by a young child is "no." They are reaching an age when they will want to decide things for themselves and sometimes this might not jell with what you want them to do. As a result, get used to hearing her say no, as well as folding her arms, pouting, and refusing to move. You may even experience her stomping her feet or making her body go rigid so that it is almost impossible for you to carry her. Believe it or not, this is a good thing. Your child is developing her own distinct personality and is beginning to want more control over her life. Although it can be stressful for parents, it is important for children to learn how to say "no" and express their own opinions.

NO TO "NO, NO, NO"

Try to keep the number of negatives you say to a minimum. At this age, toddlers get tired of hearing "no" too. Try and put a positive spin on what you say. For example, instead of saying "Don't hit the dog!" try saying "Stroke the dog softly," and then demonstrate to her how to do it.

79 "I'M NOT HAPPY—LOOK AT MY FEET."

The feet, an often overlooked part of the body, can signal whether your child may be experiencing discomfort or even pain. Most babies will wiggle or curl up when their feet are stroked or touched—it is the natural response to a tickle. Surprisingly, one of the indicators that a child is in pain is how he moves his feet. If he feels slight discomfort, your child may clench up his toes tightly. If his whole foot becomes stiff and extended toward the floor, it is likely that he is in pain.

APING APES

Believed to be a remnant of our ancestral heritage, the grasp reflex of newborn babies also occurs in the foot as baby apes cling to their mother's fur with both their hands and feet. If a finger is pressed firmly along the sole of the infant's foot the toes immediately curl tightly in an attempt to hold the finger.

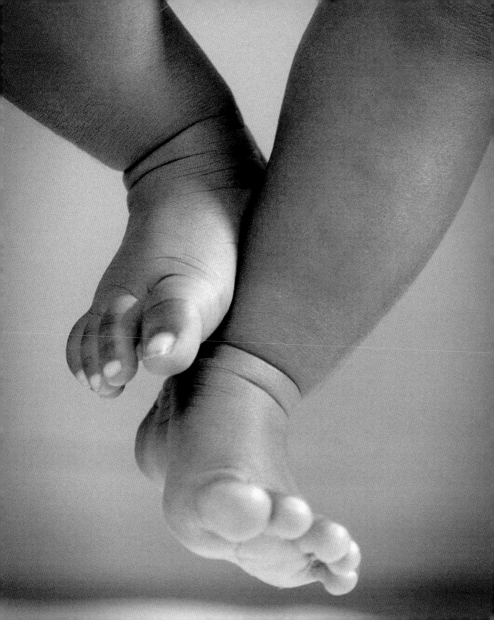

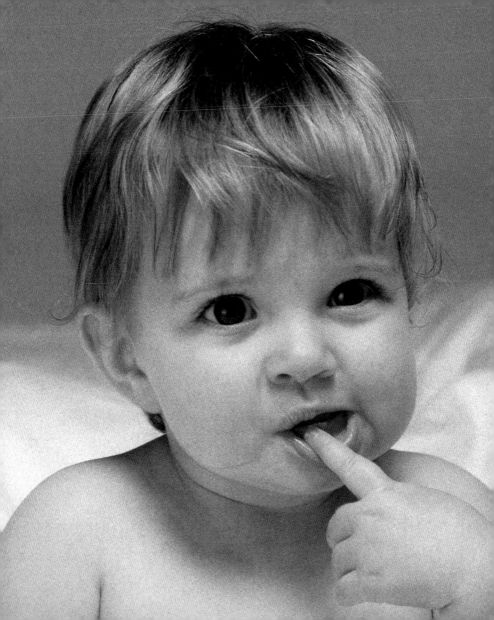

80 "OW—THEY HURT!"

Teething can be a trying time for both parents and babies alike. Often the pain of teething causes sleepless nights, anxiety, and pain. What are the signs that your child is about to cut her first tooth? Watching her body language will at least give an observant parent a heads-up on the situation and allow time for any necessary preparations. One of the first signs is chewing. Your baby will put anything in her mouth and bite down very hard. Often she will show a preference for hard or cold objects, but almost anything will do. As the teeth come closer to the surface, she will begin drooling. Sometimes the pain from the gums spreads across to the cheeks and ears. If you see her rubbing her cheeks or pulling on her ears, it is likely they are causing her discomfort.

COLD IS GOLD

There are many ways to help your child during this painful time in her life. Teething rings are useful for relieving pain, especially ones that are filled with liquid and chilled in the freezer; cold also numbs the painful gums. Cold food, such as chilled fruit puree, also helps. Failing all else, there are many teething gels available for more immediate relief.

81 "WHOA! LOOK AT THAT!"

When taking a particular interest in something, your baby's actions will point out whether it is something she has seen or heard. Children have the ability to concentrate fully on things, even to the point of blocking out all other stimuli. If a baby wants to see more of something, she will open her eyes wider and move closer to the object, as if wishing to memorize every part. If she has heard something interesting, she will lift her head and tilt her ears toward the noise. If it is a piece of music, she may even begin to tap out a rhythm with her fingers.

THAT'S GOTTA HURT

The heaviest baby ever born weighed in at an eye-watering 24 pounds. In contrast, one of the lightest babies ever born weighed just 10 ounces!

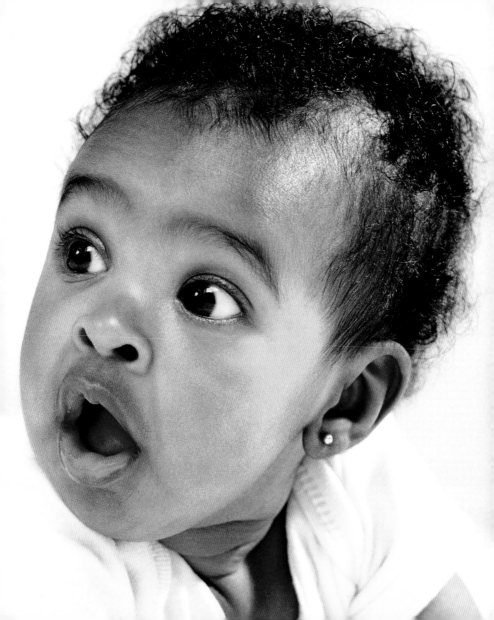

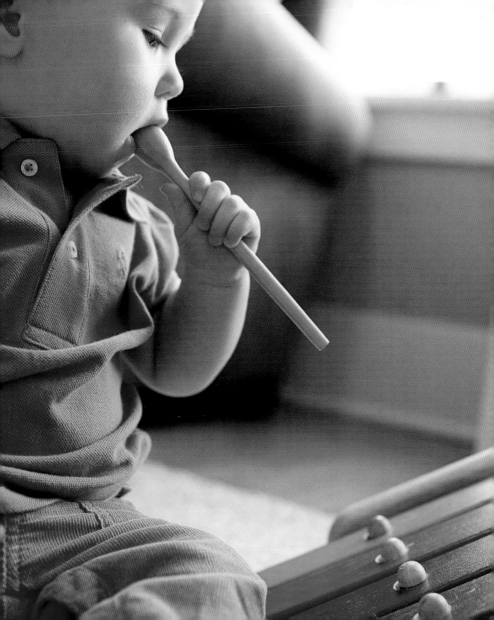

82

"I WONDER WHAT SOUND GREEN MAKES?"

Although babies can see in color from birth, they have difficulty differentiating between the different colors and shades. For example, similar colors such as red and orange are difficult to tell apart until the four-month stage. This is why a baby will pay more attention to toys or mobiles in black and white. The sharply contrasting tones grab their attention.

WITHIN THEIR REACH

At the age of four months, your baby will begin to develop depth perception, so she can tell how far away something is. Around this time, her hand-eye coordination makes an improvement—so now she can try and reach out more precisely.

83 "OKAY, I NEED A LIFT."

As babies reach nine months, hand-eye coordination starts to develop, as well as mobility and understanding. You will notice that their hand signals become clearer and easier to understand. They will convey their likes and dislikes using a mixture of gestures, expressions, and sounds. For example, should they want to be picked up, they will stretch out their arms toward you while making enthusiastic noises.

SUPERSIZE ME!

By the end of the first six months of life a baby will have doubled its original birth weight. By the end of the first year, the baby's weight will have tripled. If this state of affairs were to continue, by the time a child reached its fifth birthday it would weigh over 1,000 pounds.

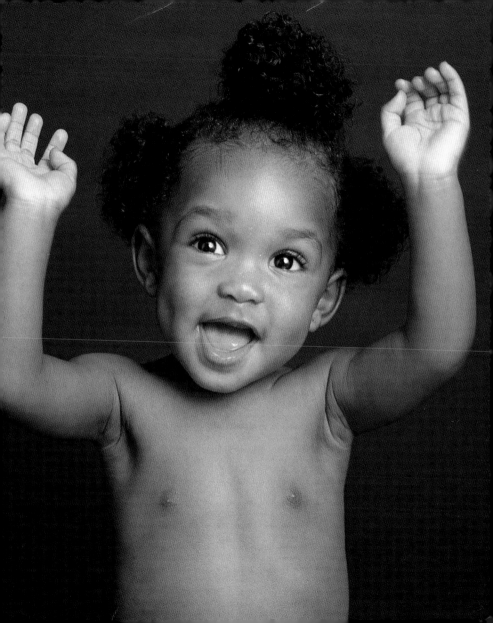

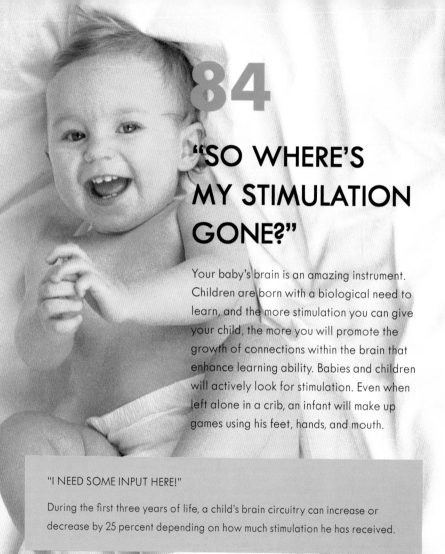

84

"SO WHERE'S MY STIMULATION GONE?"

Your baby's brain is an amazing instrument. Children are born with a biological need to learn, and the more stimulation you can give your child, the more you will promote the growth of connections within the brain that enhance learning ability. Babies and children will actively look for stimulation. Even when left alone in a crib, an infant will make up games using his feet, hands, and mouth.

"I NEED SOME INPUT HERE!"

During the first three years of life, a child's brain circuitry can increase or decrease by 25 percent depending on how much stimulation he has received.

85

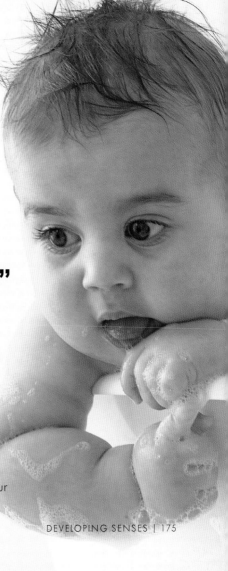

"I KNOW IT'S BATH TIME, BUT WHAT IS THAT SQUEAK?"

It is often frustrating for parents when their child doesn't seem to be paying attention to them. It is important to remember that this is not rudeness or ignorance on your child's part. It is simply their ability to focus completely on whatever they are doing by blocking out surrounding distractions. Unfortunately, this sometimes includes their parents. A gentle touch will quickly bring your child's attention back to you.

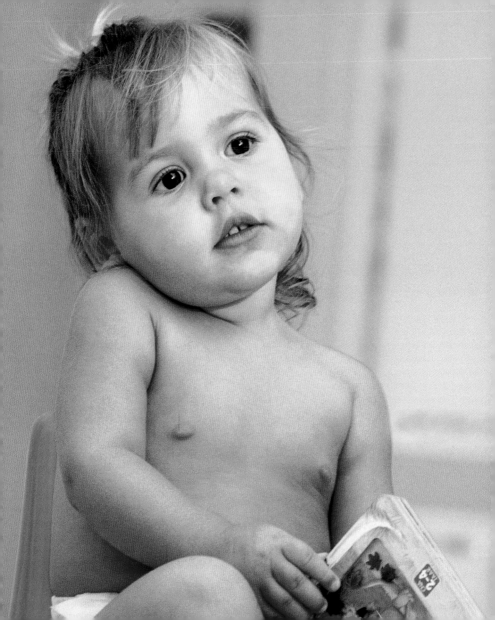

86 "THAT'S STRANGE—ANOTHER ONE ENDING 'HAPPILY EVER AFTER.'"

When younger children think about something, they are not indistinct, fuzzy thoughts, but very detailed and absorbing internal images. A baby who thinks about her mother will "see" her very clearly in her mind's eye and she will also reexperience how she feels or smells. If she has a favorite song, she will hear that tune in her head as clearly as if she were listening to the radio. Recent studies show that these moments of deep thought are a child's way of processing all the information she has absorbed during the day.

JUST REBOOTING

Parents will often notice times when their child defocuses for a few seconds while engaged in another action. Associated with these moments of quiet contemplation are some specific eye movements called "conjugolateral eye movements," also known as CLEMS.

87 "I'LL GET THE HANG OF THIS SOONER OR LATER."

As your child grows and develops confidence, you will notice times when he actively pushes you away. This usually happens when you are trying to help him with an everyday task, such as getting him dressed. Instead of being allowed to help, you are pushed aside as he tries to do it alone. Don't be upset; it is not a rejection. As he gets older, your child will want to try doing more things for himself. For parents, it is sometimes difficult to let your children attempt these little tasks because we are pressed for time or have a set routine. No matter now hard it is, allow them to try: the sense of achievement they will experience on succeeding is huge.

TOP BABY NAMES IN 1980

Girls	Boys
1 Jessica	1 Michael
2 Jennifer	2 Christopher
3 Amanda	3 Matthew
4 Ashley	4 Joshua
5 Sarah	5 David

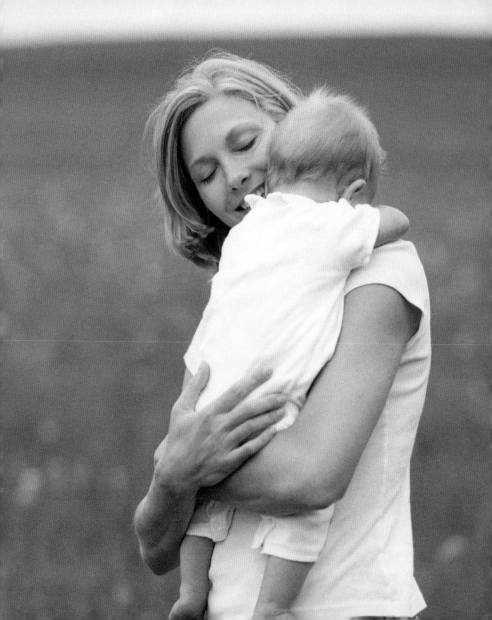

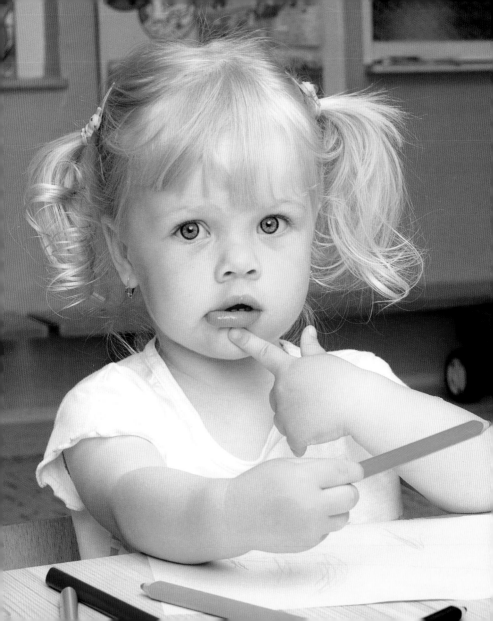

88 "I ONLY DO SHORT WORDS."

In between the ages of two and four years old, as their vocabulary begins to expand, your child may develop a stutter. Stuttering occurs when a child knows what he wants to say but cannot find just the right word. Often he will become stuck on the same word, repeating it over and over until he remembers what he wanted to say next. Sometimes there will be an elongation of the first letter in a word or he may move his mouth yet no sound comes out. Stuttering is a normal part in a child's speech development and no cause for alarm. Eighty percent of children who develop stutters will lose them by the time they reach school age.

TOP BABY NAMES IN 2017

Girls	Boys
1 Sophia	1 Jackson
2 Olivia	2 Liam
3 Emma	3 Noah
4 Ava	4 Aiden
5 Isabella	5 Lucas

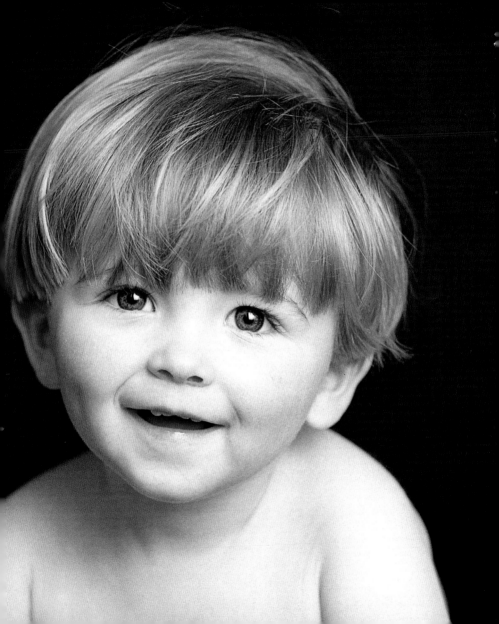

89

"GIVE ME FIVE!"

As a child grows, so will his understanding of the body language of others. One of the first things he will learn are the important "acknowledgment signals." These simple actions show you that he is listening and has understood. He will begin to nod in response to you. His smiles will become wider and more sincere as he learns to use them to express genuine pleasure rather than just mimicking your expressions. Pointing will also become an important way for him to share all his discoveries with you and show you what he wants.

YES, NO, WHAT?

Although seen as a positive action in most of the world, nodding does not always indicate a "yes." In Sri Lanka and Bulgaria, nodding actually has the opposite meaning.

90 "AND YOUR POINT IS?"

There is a reason why they are called "the terrible twos" and sometimes it will seem like your once-sweet little angel is always getting into trouble or causing you stress. It is important in times like these to try and understand the reasoning for her behavior. What you see as her being difficult, she may interpret as curiosity. For example, you may see her sticking her finger in your dog's eye. You might think she is being mean or even flirting with danger when she is really thinking something like, "I wonder what happens if I press this?" Toddlers cannot yet ask questions and, aside from sight and sound, must explore the world through touch, smell, and taste. They are intensely curious and often single-minded, but never—despite appearances to the contrary—malicious.

PIT STOP, QUICK CHANGE CHALLENGE

According to recent research, men are faster at changing diapers/nappies than women. The results show that women take, on average, two minutes and five seconds to change a diaper where men take a lightning-speed one minute and thirty-six seconds. Although, as many women already know, "faster" does not always mean "better."

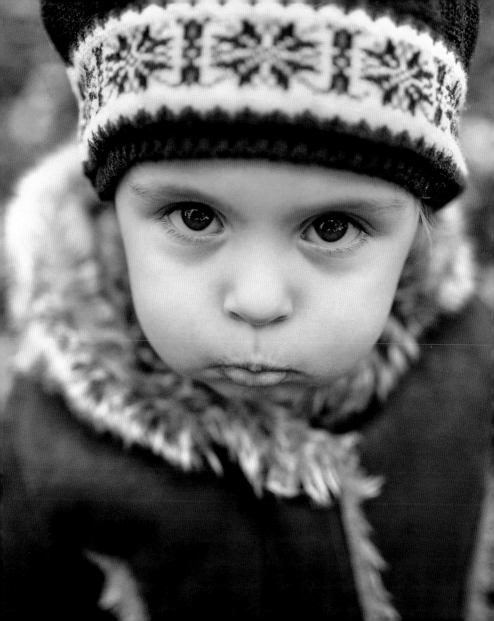

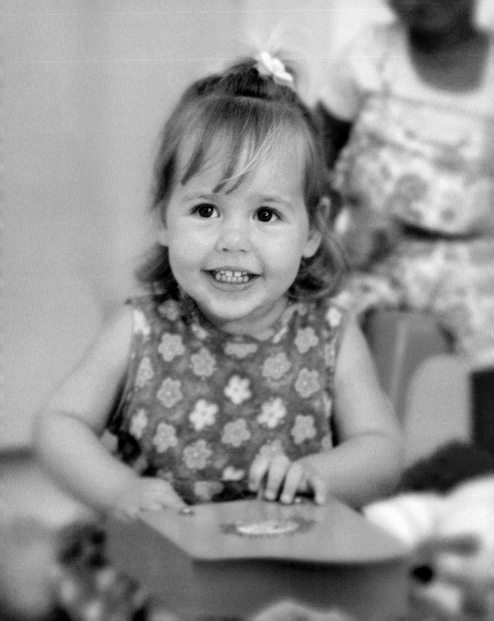

91 "I CAN PLAY IT AGAIN IF YOU LIKE."

Toddlers enjoy discovering the world a little bit at a time. You may find your toddler begins to display what looks like obsessive behavior. Perhaps she loves having the same book read to her every night, or maybe she opens and closes the same drawer over and over again with all the signs of great enjoyment. This is nothing unusual. Your child is just trying to learn about the world and trying to understand how everything works. More importantly, however, repetition is vital for toddlers because it makes them feel secure. Knowing there is something they can rely on is very soothing for a child. Demanding to hear the same story over and over helps them feel safe and gives them a sense of control.

WEIGH TO GO

Babies born during the month of May are on average seven ounces or two hundred grams heavier than those born in any other month. One quarter of the baby's total body weight is comprised of the head.

92 "DON'T TOUCH MY FAVORITE GLASS."

A toddler's love of familiarity and routine can often cause awkward situations. Sometimes it may be something as simple as only drinking from one particular bottle and refusing any alternatives. Or it could be an insistence on wearing a specific outfit every single day, all day long. If denied the object of adoration, toddlers can often become difficult, sometimes to the point of crying and tantrums. Once again, this is the child's way of dealing with the world in small, easily manageable chunks. He may not be able to drive a car, read a book, or understand a lot of what people say to him, but he can make sure he wears his tiger outfit every day or drinks from his favorite blue bottle. Such relatively tiny requirements will give him a sense of confidence and control.

IMAGINE CHRISTMAS . . .

The greatest number of babies borne by one woman is a staggering sixty-nine. A Russian woman in the eighteenth century gave birth to sixteen sets of twins, seven sets of triplets, and four sets of quadruplets.

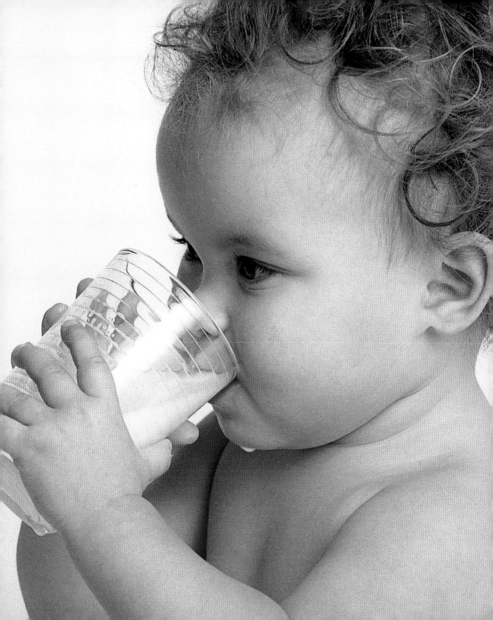

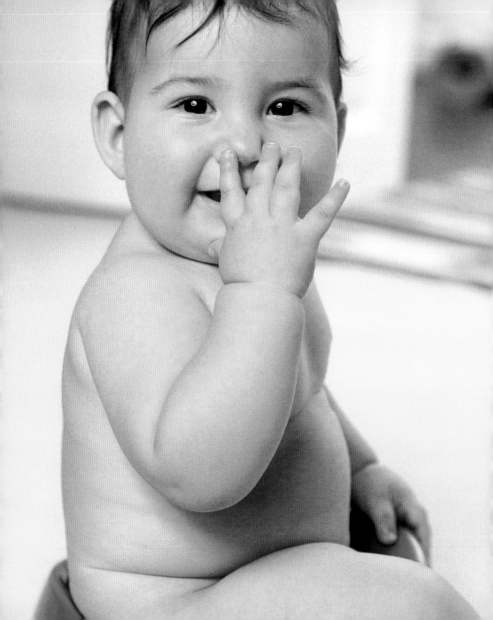

93 "OOPS! SORRY ABOUT THE SMELL."

Toilet training needn't be a daunting task for a parent or child if handled correctly. The only time it may become too stressful is if attempted before the child is ready. But how do you know when the time is right? There are clear signs you can look out for. If he becomes unhappy and uncomfortable after soiling his diaper, if he begins to concentrate while passing a stool and makes grunting noises or squats down, and if he stays dry for a couple of hours every day, he is probably ready. Also, he may begin to pay attention to you when you go to the toilet, learning through observation.

POTTY TIME

When is it not a good time to start toilet training your child? Times of stress for you and your toddler are the worst moments, such as during the arrival of a new baby or when moving to a new house.

94

"DAD. CAT. THERE. GO. NOW!"

As your child enters the toddler stage, you may notice a change in his body language. There will be differences between the body language he uses with you and that he uses with other toddlers. He will use his body to communicate directly with you, for example by pointing, touching, nodding, and shaking his head. He is using his body language in place of verbal communication. He may try to form words, although they will be difficult to understand and he may get frustrated when you cannot figure out what he is trying to say.

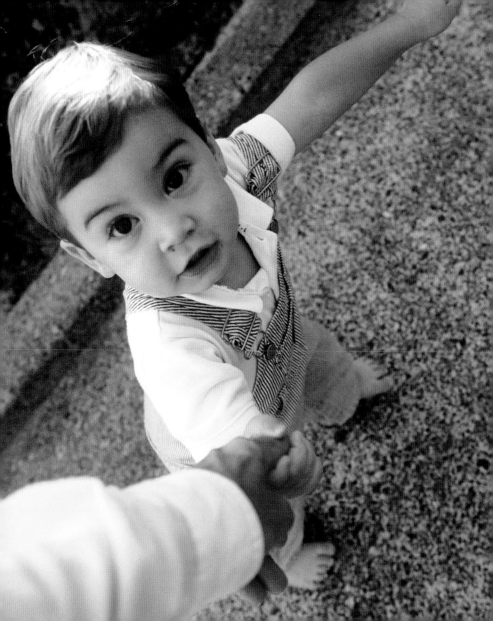

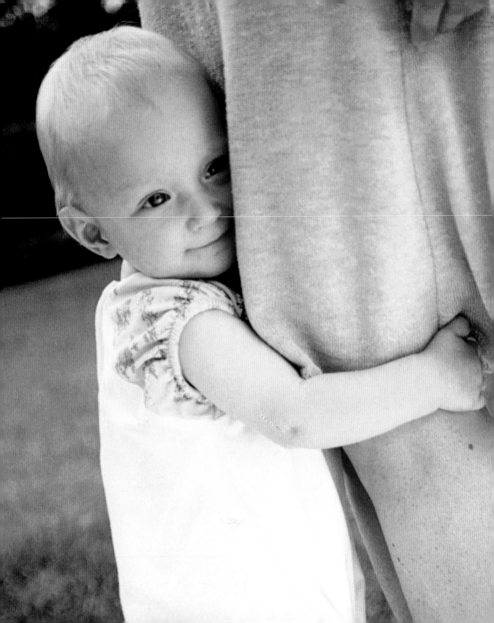

95

"DON'T MAKE ME JOIN IN!"

Reading the body language of your toddler will give you an insight into how comfortable she is in any given situation. For example, when faced with a large group of children the same age, some toddlers will react in different ways. Many will dive straight in and play happily; others may hang back and cling to their mothers. Some may even become aggressive with the other children. The comfortable and confident toddler is obviously the one happy to join in and play. The uncomfortable toddler may react with timid behavior, or go the other way and become overly aggressive.

BEETHOVEN, TOO

Scientific studies have proven that playing classical music to your children, especially Mozart, can somtimes increase your baby's intelligence.

96 "GO, YELLOW TRUCK!"

You may think your toddler is unnecessarily rough sometimes. He might throw food or toys around the room or bash the family pet. It would be easy to interpret this as aggression, but this may not be the case. Soft and gentle touches do not come naturally to toddlers, who have not yet developed control over their arm and wrist movements. Teaching your child how to be gentle will help them control their actions. Hold his hand and show him how to stroke the cat without hurting it or how to balance food on a spoon.

TWIN TRACK APPROACH

Children develop at different rates and there is no set plan to check off at certain times. This is also true of twins. Twins develop completely separately. One may be more concentrated on language, the other on movement. It is important not to compare them.

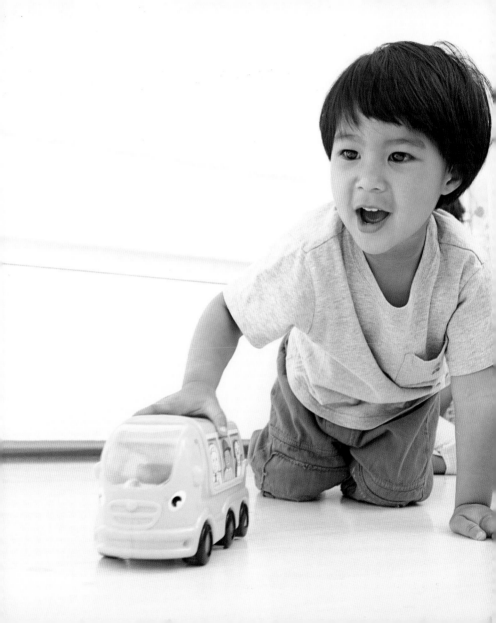

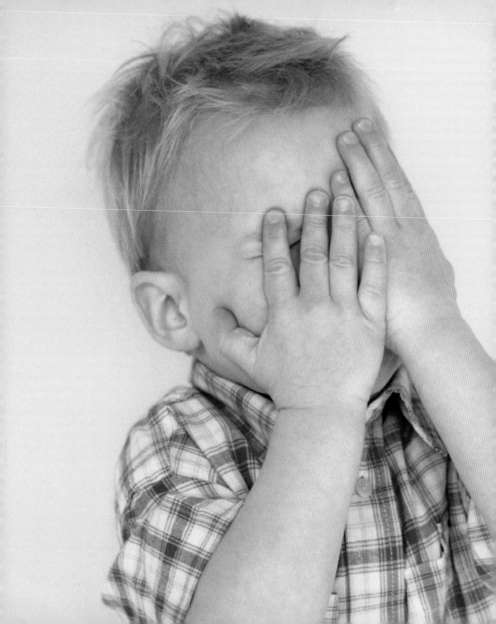

97

"OH NO—IT'S GRANDMA!"

When faced with uncertainty or something frightening, most toddlers will hold their hands in front of them, shielding their bodies. Their expressions will also reflect this fear: big wide eyes staring out of an unsmiling, serious face. This is your cue to take things slowly when introducing new and potentially frightening things—or people.

LIMIT ACCESS TO CERTAIN AREAS

Toddlers see their home as a playground and it is important to make sure it is safe. Keep medicines, cleaning products, and alcohol out of their reach. Make sure to childproof any cupboards containing dangerous materials.

98 "MOM, I SAID BOOK THE CLOWN FOR THE PARTY. NOW DEAL WITH IT."

Toddlers can be extremely sensitive. They are experiencing the world through intense emotions and limited communication skills. Their ability to talk can't keep up with all the things they want to say or ask you about. It can be extremely upsetting for them and it is up to you to try and help as much as possible. Focusing on what your child is trying to say to you is important, not just the words but the emotions behind them. If you are unsure whether or not you have grasped her meaning, then repeat what you think she said back to her, for example "You want your teddy bear?" or "You want to be carried?"

GIVE THEM YOUR ATTENTION

Make time to really connect with your child—even two minutes every half an hour is enough to increase her communication skills. When she comes to you to talk, try and give her your undivided attention. It will make her feel important and valued.

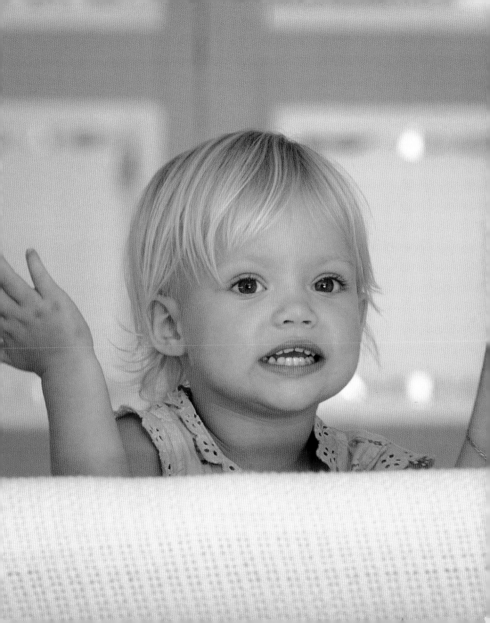

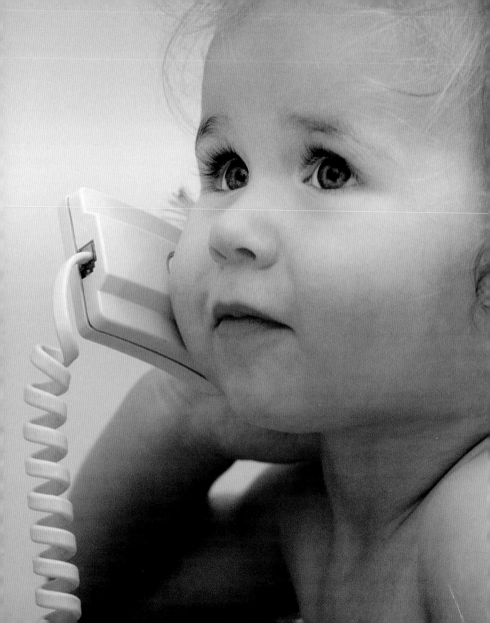

99 "OKAY, SCHEDULE THE NAP FOR TEN, AND PUT MY CALLS ON HOLD."

Toddlers can be a lot of fun, and one of the most charming things you may notice them doing is copying you. Your little cherub may sit at the computer and pretend to tap away at the keys, or simulate talking happily on the phone just like you do, or even pick up the vacuum and start cleaning the carpets. This mimicry is one of the most important ways a toddler will learn. The sense of achievement experienced by any child after completing a set task is enormous and often the praise they receive will boost their confidence even further. Such rewards will push them to try more things and copy your behavior.

LEARNING TO CARE

It is never too early to start teaching manners. Your child learns from your example, so if you want a polite child then begin by being polite to him. Say "please" when you ask him to do something and make sure you say "thank you" when he does it. Soon he will be copying your good example.

100

"I MAY BE DRESSED AS AN ANGEL, BUT I CAN BE A LITTLE DEVIL."

Beware! Not only will children copy your good behavior, but also the bad. Smokers with children will often discover their offspring holding an imaginary cigarette, pretending to smoke. Messy parents will inadvertently encourage their children to be messy, too. Perhaps most embarrassingly, if you don't watch what you say, your child may shout out an inappropriate word they have learned from you—often in a public place. Remember to be a good role model.

"The toddler must say 'no' in order to find out who she is. The adolescent says 'no' to assert who she is not."
Louise Kaplan

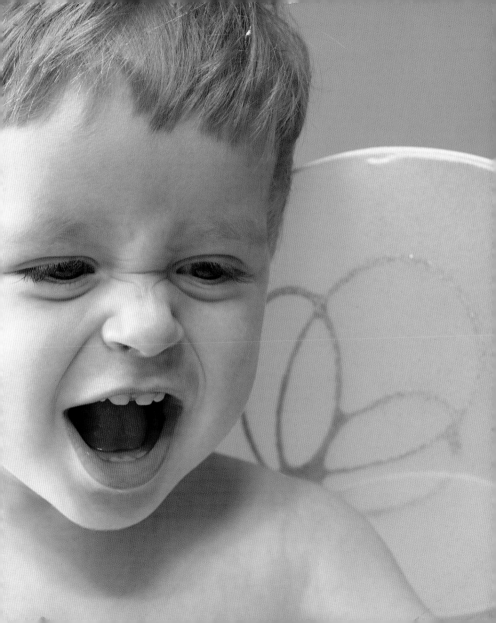

Index

Acknowledgments

I would like to thank my three children, Maia, Bethany, and Sam, for their contribution to this project. The practical insight into the minds of youngsters was invaluable in writing the book. I couldn't have written it without them. They teach me something new every day. I would also like to thank my parents for providing a perfect model in parenting, which I hope to live up to. Thanks also go to the many wonderful children of Southdown school in Wales who first inspired my interest in child psychology, and to the teachers who showed such patience, wisdom, and kindness.